O U
OXFORD UROLOGY LIBRARY

Overactive Bladder Syndrome and Urinary Incontinence

Edited by

Dr Hashim Hashim

Consultant Urological Surgeon,
Bristol Urological Institute, Southmead Hospital,
Bristol, UK

Professor Paul Abrams

Bristol Urological Institute, Southmead Hospital,
Bristol, UK

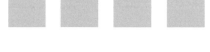

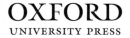

OXFORD
UNIVERSITY PRESS

OXFORD
UNIVERSITY PRESS

Great Clarendon Street, Oxford OX2 6DP

Oxford University Press is a department of the University of Oxford.
It furthers the University's objective of excellence in research, scholarship,
and education by publishing worldwide in

Oxford New York

Auckland Cape Town Dar es Salaam Hong Kong Karachi
Kuala Lumpur Madrid Melbourne Mexico City Nairobi
New Delhi Shanghai Taipei Toronto

With offices in

Argentina Austria Brazil Chile Czech Republic France Greece
Guatemala Hungary Italy Japan Poland Portugal Singapore
South Korea Switzerland Thailand Turkey Ukraine Vietnam

Oxford is a registered trade mark of Oxford University Press
in the UK and in certain other countries

Published in the United States
by Oxford University Press Inc., New York

British Library Cataloguing in Publication Data

Data available

Library of Congress Cataloging in Publication Data

Data available

Typeset by Glyph International, Bangalore, India
Printed in Great Britain on acid-free paper by
Ashford Colour Press Ltd, Gosport, Hampshire

ISBN 978–0–19–959939–4

10 9 8 7 6 5 4 3 2 1

Whilst every effort has been made to ensure that the contents of this book
are as complete, accurate and-up-to-date as possible at the date of writing.
Oxford University Press is not able to give any guarantee or assurance that
such is the case. Readers are urged to take appropriately qualified medical
advice in all cases. The information in this book is intended to be useful to
the general reader, but should not be used as a means of self-diagnosis or
for the prescription of medication.

Contents

Preface

Overactive bladder (OAB) syndrome and urinary incontinence (UI) are prevalent conditions affecting all age groups. However, they are often neglected by health care professionals as they do not cause mortality. On the other hand, the morbidity and effect on quality of life from OAB and UI can be very drastic for the individual. These subjects are often not taught at medical school or during residency training. Both OAB and UI tend to be managed by specialists, with expertise in lower urinary tract dysfunction, while in fact the majority of cases can be initially managed in the primary care setting.

This book is written by experts in the field, with residents, trainees, primary care physicians and allied health-care professionals in mind. It is clinically orientated and covers all aspects of OAB and UI from definitions to management of complex cases. However the text is not exhaustive and the appendix at the end of the book includes useful easy-to-follow guidelines. The book is pocket-sized and easy to read.

We would like to extend our sincere thanks to the authors who have participated in the book and also to the publishers Oxford University Press for their work on the book. Finally, we would like to thank our families for bearing with us while the book was being written.

Hashim Hashim
Paul Abrams

Foreword

'Overactive bladder syndrome and urinary incontinence' is a valuable handbook which covers the important aspects of overactive bladder (OAB) syndrome and urinary incontinence (UI). It is divided into sections which cover definitions, epidemiology, pathophysiology, assessment and treatment of OAB and urinary incontinence. The last chapter addresses the management of complex cases such as post-prostatectomy incontinence and mixed urinary incontinence. The appendix includes guidelines from the International consultation on urological diseases and the National Institute of Health and Clinical Excellence in the UK.

The authors are all experts in the field of OAB and incontinence and have taken every effort to make the book flow in a clinically relevant manner that is applicable to everyday practice. The book is aimed at trainees, general practitioners, allied health-care providers and general urologists and urogynaecologists. It is easy to carry around and its pocket-size which makes it ideal for every health-care professional's briefcase or pocket who deals with patients that have OAB and UI.

Alan J. Wein, MD, PhD (hon),
Professor & Chair, Division of Urology,
University of Pennsylvania Health System,
Philadelphia, PA, USA

Symbols and abbreviations

5ARI	5-alpha reductase inhibitor
Ach	Acetylcholine
ADLs	Activities of daily living
AR	Adrenoceptor
AUS	Artificial urinary sphincter
BOO	Bladder outlet obstruction
BoTN	Botulinum toxin
BTA	Botulinum toxin A
CMG	Cystometrogram
DHIC	Detrusor hyperactivity with impaired contractility
DLPP	Detrusor leak point pressure
DO	Detrusor overactivity
DOI	Detrusor overactivity incontinence
DRE	Digital rectal examination
DRG	Dorsal root ganglia
EMG	Electromyography
ES	Electrical stimulation
FDA	Food and Drug Administration
FVC	Frequency-volume chart
ICI	International Consultation on Incontinence
IPG	Impulse generator
ICIQ	ICI Questionnaire
ICS	International Continence Society
ICUD	International Consultation on Urological Diseases
ISC	Intermittent self-catheterization
LUT	Lower urinary tract
LUTS	Lower urinary tract symptoms
mg	Milligram
mL	Millilitres
MMK	Marshall-Marchetti-Krantz
MRI	Magnetic resonance imaging

MUI	Mixed urinary incontinence
NE	Norepinephrine
NICE	National Institute for Health and Clinical Excellence
OAB	Overactive bladder syndrome
OXY-IR	Oxybutynin immediate-release
PAG	Periaqueductal grey
PFMT	Pelvic floor muscle training
PFS	Pressure-flow studies
PMC	Pontine micturition centre
POP	Pelvic organ prolapse
PPI	Post-prostatectomy incontinence
PRB	Pressure-regulating balloon
PSA	Prostate specific antigen
Pt	Patient
PTNS	Percutaneous tibial nerve stimulation
PUL	Pubo-urethral ligaments
PVR	Post-void residual
Qol	Quality of life
Rx	Treatment
RTX	Resiniferatoxin
SNS	Sacral nerve stimulation
SUI	Stress urinary incontinence
TCA	Tricyclic antidepressants
TENS	Transcutaneous electrical nerve stimulation
TVT	Transvaginal tape
UI	Urinary incontinence
USI	Urodynamic stress incontinence
UT	Upper tract
UTI	Urinary tract infection
UUI	Urgency urinary incontinence
VLPP	Valsalva leak point pressure

Contributors

Professor Paul Abrams
Bristol Urological Institute,
Bristol, UK

Professor Roger R. Dmochowski
Vanderbilt University,
Tennessee, USA

Dr Alexander Gomelsky
LSUHSC-Shreveport,
Department of Urology,
LA, USA

Dr Hashim Hashim
Consultant Urological Surgeon,
Bristol Urological Institute,
Southmead Hospital,
Bristol, UK

Dr W. Stuart Reynolds
Department of Urology,
Vanderbilt University Medical
Center, Nashville, USA

Chapter 1

Definition of overactive bladder syndrome and stress urinary incontinence

Hashim Hashim & Paul Abrams

> **Key points**
>
> - Overactive bladder (OAB) syndrome is a symptom complex consisting of urinary urgency, with or without urgency urinary incontinence, usually accompanied by frequency and nocturia, in the absence of urinary tract infection or other obvious pathology.
> - Urinary incontinence (UI) is the complaint of involuntary loss of urine.
> - Urgency urinary incontinence (UUI) is the complaint of involuntary loss of urine associated with urgency.
> - Stress urinary incontinence (SUI) is the complaint of involuntary loss of urine on effort or physical exertion including sporting activities, or on sneezing or coughing.

1.1 Lower urinary tract symptoms

Over the past 10 years there have been new definitions of lower urinary tract symptoms. It is therefore important that all health-care professionals speak the same language and hence this chapter is very important in setting the rest of the book in the context of standardized terminology.

Lower urinary tract symptoms can be divided into three main groups: storage symptoms, voiding symptoms, and post-micturition symptoms.

Storage symptoms occur when the bladder is filling with urine. These have previously been known as 'irritative' symptoms. Voiding symptoms occur when the person is voiding. In men, these used to be known as 'prostatism' or 'prostatic symptoms'. Post-micturition

Table 1.1 Lower urinary tract symptoms		
Storage	**Voiding**	**Post-micturition**
• Urgency • Frequency • Nocturia • Incontinence	• Hesitancy • Straining • Spraying • Poor stream • Dysuria • Intermittency	• Feeling of incomplete bladder emptying • Post-micturition dribble

symptoms occur after voiding. Table 1.1 above shows the symptoms that occur with each group. This chapter and book will concentrate on the storage symptoms.

1.2 Urinary incontinence

Urinary incontinence (UI) is the complaint of any involuntary loss (leakage) of urine. The two main types of incontinence are stress urinary incontinence (SUI) and urgency urinary incontinence (UUI). When the patient complains of both types of incontinence, they are said to have mixed urinary incontinence (MUI).

SUI is the complaint of involuntary loss of urine on effort or physical exertion including sporting activities or on sneezing or coughing. In other words, it is activity-related incontinence. This used to be called 'genuine stress incontinence'. If a patient leaks during urodynamics on coughing, straining or any activity, this is now termed urodynamic stress incontinence (USI).

UUI is the complaint of involuntary loss of urine associated with urgency. It may be accompanied by or immediately preceded by urgency.

Other types of incontinence have also been described and include postural urinary incontinence (associated with change in body position), enuresis (occurs during sleep), continuous urinary incontinence, insensible (unconscious) urinary incontinence (feeling of wetness with no provocative cause), and coital urinary incontinence.

1.3 Overactive bladder syndrome

Overactive bladder (OAB) syndrome is a symptom complex consisting of urinary urgency, with or without urgency urinary incontinence, usually accompanied by frequency and nocturia, in the absence of urinary tract infections or other obvious pathology. It has also been known as urgency-frequency syndrome. Urgency is

Table 1.2 Symptoms of OAB
Urgency is the complaint of a sudden compelling desire to pass urine, which is difficult to defer. This essentially means that when the patient has to go to void, they have to go.
Daytime urinary frequency is the complaint that micturition occurs more frequently than previously deemed normal. This used to be defined as eight or more voids but now is more subjective and depends on whether the patient feels that they are going more often to void.
Nocturia is the complaint that the individual has to wake up at night one or more times to void. Each void is preceded and followed by sleep.
Urgency urinary incontinence is the complaint of involuntary leakage of urine which is accompanied by or immediately preceded by urgency.

the key symptom and the driving force of OAB; however, we still do not have an adequately validated tool to measure urgency. Table 1.2 above defines these terms.

It is important to realize that the definition of OAB is based on a clinical diagnosis and complements previous definitions which were based on abnormal detrusor function during the filling phase of cystometry. If someone has OAB, then this is suggestive of uro-dynamically demonstrable detrusor overactivity (DO), which may be spontaneous or provoked. DO can be further sub-classified into idiopathic or neurogenic. DO is defined as urodynamically demon-strable involuntary detrusor contractions during filling cystometry. The term DO is now used instead of the old term 'detrusor instability'. If a patient leaks during filling cystometry while having a detrusor over-activity wave, this is called detrusor overactivity incontinence (DOI).

Not all patients with OAB will have DO nor will all patients with DO have OAB. In one series, 82% of men with OAB had DO and 58% of women with OAB had DO.

Key references

Abrams P, Cardozo L, Fall M, Griffiths D, Rosier P, Ulmsten U, *et al.* (2002). The standardisation of terminology of lower urinary tract function: report from the Standardisation Sub-committee of the International Continence Society. *Neurourol Urodyn*, **21**, 167–78.

Haylen BT, De Ridder D, Freeman RM, Swift SE, Berghmans B, Lee J, *et al.* (2010). An International Urogynecological Association (IUGA)/International Continence Society (ICS) joint report on the terminology for female pelvic floor dysfunction. *Neurourol Urodyn*, **29**, 4–20.

Hashim H, Abrams P (2006). Is the bladder a reliable witness for predicting detrusor overactivity? *J Urol*, **175**, 191–4.

Chapter 2

Epidemiology of overactive bladder syndrome and urinary incontinence

Hashim Hashim & Paul Abrams

Key points

- Overactive bladder (OAB) syndrome and urinary incontinence (UI) are prevalent conditions.
- Storage lower urinary tract symptoms (LUTS) are more prevalent than voiding or post-micturition LUTS.
- Prevalence of OAB and UI:
  - increases with age
  - is slightly higher in women than men
  - varies by country
  - is higher than many other co-morbidities or chronic conditions.
- OAB and UI negatively affect quality of life.
- OAB and UI cost society millions of dollars.

2.1 Urinary incontinence

2.1.1 Prevalence

The prevalence of urinary incontinence (UI) is difficult to quantify and several studies report different results in women ranging between 5 and 69%. It is even more difficult to quote the prevalence based on type of incontinence. This is because of the different definitions, population samples, age ranges and questionnaires used.

In women, the prevalence is almost equally distributed between the three types of incontinence with 34% mixed urinary incontinence (MUI), 34% stress urinary incontinence (SUI) and 32% urgency urinary incontinence (UUI). What is known is that the prevalence of SUI is higher in young and middle-aged women, and that older women are more likely to have MUI and UUI. Women are at least twice more likely to have UI than men.

There are also variations in prevalence between different countries. White, non-Hispanic women tend to have a substantially higher prevalence of SUI than Black or Asian women, for no apparent reasons.

Body mass, pregnancy, labour, and vaginal delivery are risk factors for SUI in women. Other potential risk factors, including smoking, diet, depression, constipation, urinary tract infections, and exercise, have not been established as aetiological risk factors.

The prevalence of UI in men has not been as widely studied as in women, but has been reported to be between 1 and 39%. UUI is the most predominant type ranging between 40 and 80%. It is followed by MUI (10–30%), and then SUI (<10%).

Risk factors for UI in men include increasing age, presence of LUTS, urinary tract infections, functional and cognitive impairment, neurological disorders, and prostatectomy.

It is estimated that 346 million individuals worldwide had UI in 2008, and this is expected to rise to 383 million in 2013 and 420 million in 2018.

2.1.2 **Cost**

To date, no studies have looked at the costs of UI by type. Costs include direct care costs, such as laundry, pads and medications, and indirect costs, such as loss of productivity, and the cost of consequences, such as urinary tract infections, falls, and fractures. These costs will be borne by society, which includes the patient and family, the government, and the health providers.

In the US, the direct health-care costs for UI in 1995 were estimated to be $16.3 billion per year. This rose to US$19.5 billion in 2000, with $14.2 billion being borne by community residents and $5.3 billion by institutional residents.

In 2000, the UK direct cost of clinically significant storage symptoms, borne by the health service, was estimated to be £536 million (£233 million for women) and by individuals to be £207 million (£178 million for women). The indirect costs borne by individuals were estimated to be £669 million (£368 million for women). This gives a total annual cost of £1.41 billion, amounting to about 1.1% of the National Health Service expenditure.

2.2 **Overactive bladder**

2.2.1 **Prevalence**

The overall prevalence of OAB is about 12%, being slightly higher in women compared with men. In adult males, prevalence varies from

10.2 to 17.4%, and in females from 7.7 to 31.3%, depending on the definition used. Even though OAB is prevalent, only 60% of sufferers actually seek medical advice and, of those, only 27% receive any treatment.

OAB is more common in men than women after the age of 60 and more common in women than men below the age of 60. Prevalence also varies slightly between countries, being highest in Sweden, when compared with four other countries, which may be due to cultural differences or even possibly due to differences in the weather as Sweden has a colder climate than the other countries included in the studies. It is our impression, from clinical practice, that patients' symptoms of OAB are much better during the summer compared with the winter, possibly due to sweating, which is likely to reduce urine production but also partly due to a decrease in the consumption of hot caffeine-containing drinks, such as tea and coffee. Also, cold weather may be provocative for detrusor overactivity.

It is estimated that 455 million individuals worldwide had OAB in 2008, and this is expected to rise to 500 million in 2013 and 545 million in 2018.

2.2.2 Cost

Not only is OAB a prevalent condition, but it can also have significant impact on the individual's quality of life (QoL) and leads to significant costs to society. In sufferers, OAB can significantly affect all aspects of QoL including social, psychological, occupational, domestic, physical, and sexual aspects. In one study, over 21% of the population were worried about interrupting meetings due to frequent trips to the toilet, and 3% of the population changed jobs or were fired because of their bladder control problems. In fact, it has been found that OAB has a greater impact on QoL than diabetes. Unfortunately, many sufferers do not present to the healthcare provider, thus OAB remains under-reported, despite increased awareness, and improved diagnosis and treatment.

Patients with OAB tend to visit the toilet more often, have an increased risk of urinary tract infections, and twice the odds of being injured in a fall with an increased risk of fractures, especially in the elderly, who may have to rush to the toilet to void when they suffer an urgency episode, and on the way to the toilet, end up falling and fracturing a limb. Overall, patients with UUI have a 30% increased risk of falls and 3% increased risk of fractures. About 30% of patients reported that having OAB symptoms made them feel depressed, and 28% reported feeling very stressed. Those with UUI had more emotional stress (36 vs 20%) and depression (40 vs 23%) than those with urgency, but without UUI.

It can be easily seen that if all these problems affect individuals, and if they were added together, they will significantly increase the costs to society. It has been estimated, in the USA, that OAB in 2000 was costing about $12.6 billion per year ranking fifth after arthritis, incontinence, pneumonia/influenza and osteoporosis. In 2007, these costs were estimated to be $65.9 billion in total national costs, with costs predicted to rise to $76.2 billion in 2015 and then to $82.6 billion in 2020. These costs are comparable to the costs of each of asthma and osteoporosis.

In Europe, the direct cost of OAB in 2000 was estimated at €4.2 billion across five European countries and this was projected to increase to €5.2 billion by 2020. This worked out as an annual cost of €269–706 per patient per year and consisted largely of incontinence pads. This is probably an underestimate as these data were based on a study conducted about 10 years ago and with an ageing population these figures will probably be higher and these are only the direct costs. The societal costs will probably be much higher.

Key references

Abrams P, Kelleher CJ, Kerr LA, Rogers RG (2000). Overactive bladder significantly affects quality of life. *Am J Manag Care,* **6**, 580–90.

Chiaffarino F, Parazzini F, Lavezzari M, Giambanco V (2003). Impact of urinary incontinence and overactive bladder on quality of life. *Eur Urol,* **43**, 535–38.

Ganz ML, Smalarz AM, Krupski TL, Anger JT, Hu JC, Wittrup-Jensen KU, *et al.* (2010). Economic costs of overactive bladder in the United States. *Urology,* **75**, 526–32.

Hannestad YS, Rortveit G, Daltveit AK, Hunskaar S (2003). Are smoking and other lifestyle factors associated with female urinary incontinence? The Norwegian EPINCONT Study. *Br J Obstet Gynecol,* **110**, 247–54.

Hu TW, Wagner TH, Bentkover JD, Leblanc K, Zhou SZ, Hunt T (2004). Costs of urinary incontinence and overactive bladder in the United States: a comparative study. *Urology,* **63**, 461–65.

Irwin DE, Milsom I, Hunskaar S, Reilly K, Kopp Z, Herschorn S, *et al.* (2006a). Population-based survey of urinary incontinence, overactive bladder, and other lower urinary tract symptoms in five countries: results of the EPIC study. *Eur Urol,* **50**, 1306–14.

Irwin DE, Milsom I, Kopp Z, Abrams P, Cardozo L (2006b). Impact of overactive bladder symptoms on employment, social interactions and emotional well-being in six European countries. *Br J Urol Int,* **97**, 96–100.

Liberman JN, Hunt TL, Stewart WF, Wein A, Zhou Z, Herzog AR, *et al.* (2001). Health-related quality of life among adults with symptoms of overactive bladder: results from a U.S. community-based survey. *Urology,* **57**, 1044–50.

Milsom I, Abrams P, Cardozo L, Roberts RG, Thuroff J, Wein AJ (2001). How widespread are the symptoms of an overactive bladder and how are they managed? A population-based prevalence study. *Br J Urol Int,* **87**, 760–66.

Reeves P, Irwin D, Kelleher C, Milsom I, Kopp Z, Calvert N, *et al.* (2006). The current and future burden and cost of overactive bladder in five European countries. *Eur Urol,* **50**, 1050–57.

Stewart WF, Van Rooyen JB, Cundiff GW, Abrams P, Herzog AR, Corey R, *et al.* (2003). Prevalence and burden of overactive bladder in the United States. *World J Urol,* **20**, 327–36.

Inwin DE, Kopp ZS, Agatep B, Milsom I, Abrams P (2011). Worldwide prevalence estimates of lower uinary tract symptoms, overactive bladder, urinary incontinence and bladder outlet obstruction. *BJU Int* (Epub ahead of print).

Chapter 3

Theories behind overactive bladder syndrome and stress urinary incontinence

Alexander Gomelsky & Roger R. Dmochowski

> **Key points**
>
> - Efficient urinary storage requires co-operation between the bladder, urethra, pelvic musculature, and peripheral and central nerve centres.
> - Three sets of efferent nerves (sympathetic, parasympathetic, and somatic) are responsible for bladder relaxation and outlet contraction during urinary storage.
> - Mechanisms contributing to overactive bladder symptoms may be sensory or motor, and may be neurogenic, myogenic, mixed, or idiopathic in origin.
> - Stress urinary incontinence results from a lack of urethral coaptation, a defect in support by the external sphincter or pelvic floor musculature, or both.

3.1 Introduction

The fourth International Consultation on Incontinence (ICI) recently redefined the signs and symptoms associated with lower urinary tract symptoms (LUTS). The symptoms of LUTS were categorized into several distinct types of incontinence (see Chapter 1).

Overactive bladder (OAB) is a result of a complex interaction between the bladder, neurotransmitters, and peripheral and central nerve centres. Likewise, stress urinary incontinence (SUI) may also be multifactorial in aetiology. To understand the theories behind the pathophysiology of incontinence, it is important to understand the normal anatomy and physiology of the urinary tract. The pathophysiology of urinary incontinence follows. For conciseness, this chapter will be devoted only to OAB, urgency urinary incontinence (UUI) and SUI.

3.2 **Anatomy of the lower urinary tract**

3.2.1 **Bladder**

The bladder is composed of several layers and each is integral to its function. The mucosa (superficial to deep) consists of an epithelium, a lamina propria, and a basal membrane.

- The epithelium is rugated when the bladder is empty and becomes smooth and flat when the bladder is distended with urine
- The most superficial of the three to six layers of the 'urothelium' is lined with specialized, hexagonal transitional (umbrella) cells
- There is an intermediate layer and the deepest epithelial layer is a basal cell layer attached to a thin basement membrane.

The umbrella cells are interconnected by tight junctions that minimize the unregulated movement of ions and solutes between cells, while proteins found on the apical surface of the umbrella cells reduce the permeability of the cells to small molecules, such as water, urea, and protons. Thus, the epithelial barrier is able to retain urine inside the bladder lumen while preventing the passage of ions, solutes, and toxins into deeper layers of the epithelium and detrusor muscle. Additionally, the urothelium may play a role in normal bladder function and OAB.

Deep to the basement membrane, the lamina propria forms a thick layer of fibro-elastic connective tissue that distends significantly during bladder filling. The lamina propria contains blood vessels, interstitial cells, and extracellular matrix. The bladder muscle (detrusor) lies beneath the lamina propria, and is composed of large smooth muscle fibres loosely arranged into three layers. The large, branching, interlacing bundles composing the external and internal layers are longitudinally arranged, while the middle layer is circular. These muscle layers are not distinct at the lateral and upper aspects of the bladder. At the bladder neck, the large smooth muscle bundles seen in the remainder of the bladder are replaced by finer fibres. In women, the inner longitudinal smooth muscle fibres converge and extend caudally as the inner longitudinal layer of the urethra.

3.2.2 **Bladder outlet/urethra**

The epithelial lining of the female urethra changes gradually from transitional epithelium to non-keratinized squamous epithelium distally. A thick submucosa supports the epithelium and peri-urethral glands. At rest, well-vascularized, submucosal connective tissue compresses urethral mucosal folds to create a watertight seal. Luminal secretions from the peri-urethral glands increase urethral wall tension and further augment the urethral seal. In women, the mucosa and submucosa are oestrogen dependent and may atrophy with oestrogen depletion.

A thick layer of inner longitudinal smooth muscle extends from the bladder to the external meatus. The intrinsic urethral (smooth) sphincter is normally closed at rest, with layers of detrusor muscle and elastin contributing to static compression. A thin layer of circular smooth muscle wraps around the longitudinal fibres over the entire length of the urethra.

The extrinsic sphincter is the outer layer of the urethra and is composed of circularly-arranged bundles of striated muscle. This sphincter is thickest ventrally and sparse dorsally, like the smooth muscle layers. The extrinsic sphincter is composed of two physiologically distinct components:

- The inner (paraurethral) layer of striated muscle is composed of slow-twitch muscle fibres which maintain tonic contraction of the urethra and may be important in passive continence
- The outer (peri-urethral) layer consists of fast-twitch fibres and is similar to the surrounding levator ani musculature. This muscle layer attaches to the urethra only on the posterior aspect and appears to be important during stress manoeuvres.

3.2.3 **Pelvic floor musculature**
The pelvic muscles and fasciae are under a state of tonic contraction and work together to prevent urinary incontinence and pelvic prolapse. There are three key supportive elements:

- Distally, the pubovisceral and perineal muscles form a sphincter around the urogenital hiatus. This includes the pubourethral ligament that forms a sling that suspends the urethra under the pubic symphysis
- The levator plate acts as a horizontal shelf under the bladder, cervix, posterior vagina, and rectum
- Proximally, the cardinal and uterosacral ligaments anchor the pelvic organs over the levator plate.

3.2.4 **Peripheral innervation**
The lower urinary tract is innervated by three sets of efferent peripheral nerves involving the sympathetic, parasympathetic, and somatic nervous systems.

Sympathetic
Sympathetic preganglionic outflow emerges from the lumbar spinal cord and passes in sequence to the lumbosacral sympathetic chain

ganglia, inferior splanchnic nerves, and prevertebral inferior mesenteric ganglia. Pre- and post-ganglionic sympathetic axons travel in the hypogastric nerve to the pelvic plexus and to the bladder neck and proximal urethra. Sympathetic efferent pathways in the hypogastric and pelvic nerves inhibit detrusor smooth muscle through β-adrenoceptors and stimulate smooth muscle in the bladder neck and proximal urethra through α_1-adrenoceptors. The end result is urinary storage by detrusor inhibition and urethral contraction.

Parasympathetic

Parasympathetic preganglionic axons originate in the sacral spinal cord and pass via the pelvic nerve to postganglionic neurons in the pelvic plexus and detrusor. Parasympathetic preganglionic neurons release the excitatory neurotransmitter acetylcholine (Ach) at peripheral ganglia. This is mediated by muscarinic receptors. Transmission in bladder ganglia is mediated by a nicotinic cholinergic mechanism that may be modulated by muscarinic, adrenergic, purinergic, and peptidergic receptors. The end result is bladder contraction and relaxation of the bladder outlet to promote urinary emptying.

Somatic

Sacral somatic pathways originate in Onuf's nucleus and are contained in the pudendal nerve, which provides innervation to the striated urethral sphincter and pelvic floor musculature. Ach is the neurotransmitter which stimulates post-junctional nicotinic receptors after release.

Afferent innervation

Sensory axons in the pelvic, hypogastric, and pudendal nerves transmit information from the lower urinary tract to the lumbosacral spinal cord. The primary afferent neurons of the pelvic and pudendal nerves are contained in sacral dorsal root ganglia (DRG), whereas afferent neurons of the hypogastric nerves originate in the rostral lumbar DRG. The central axons of the DRG neurons carry the sensory information from the lower urinary tract to second-order neurons in the spinal cord mainly via the pelvic nerve. Finely-myelinated (Aδ) axons originate in the detrusor and sense bladder fullness via increasing wall tension. When the bladder is distended, Aδ fibres increase firing and initiate the micturition reflex. During inflammation, these axons increase their discharge at a lower pressure threshold. Unmyelinated (C) fibres are located within the bladder smooth muscle where they innervate the basal urothelium, and in the mucosa, where they respond to stretch via bladder volume sensors. Detrusor C-fibres increase dramatically in density as they approach the bladder neck and proximal urethra. Like Aδ axons, these axons may increase their discharge at a lower pressure threshold during times of inflammation. C-fibres found in the mucosa

Index

Please note that page references to flowcharts or tables will be in *italic* print

may be nociceptive to overdistention and may be very sensitive to bladder irritation.

3.2.5 Central innervation

Afferent input from the bladder and urethra travels in the pelvic nerve and synapses in the sacral spinal cord. Input then ascends through the spinal cord to the peri-aqueductal grey (PAG) of the pons. The PAG, in turn, provides input to the pontine micturition centre (PMC). Descending input from the PMC provides input to parasympathetic motor neurons in the sacral spinal cord and Onuf's nucleus.

3.3 Physiology of normal urinary storage

The outcome of efficient urinary storage is retention of a socially acceptable amount of urine at a low bladder pressure and a competent and closed bladder outlet, in the absence of detrusor overactivity (DO):

- The accommodation of urine (compliance) is primarily a passive phenomenon dependent on the intrinsic properties and collagen content of the detrusor and the quiescence of the parasympathetic pathway. Urinary storage is achieved mainly by spinal reflex pathways which are under supraspinal control via the PAG and the PMC
- Increased wall tension during filling activates bladder afferent nerves (through $A\delta$ axons in the pelvic nerve), activating several efferent pathways
- Contraction of the external sphincter and pelvic floor striated musculature via the pudendal nerve (nicotinic receptor)
- Internal sphincter contraction (α_1-adrenoceptors) and ganglionic inhibition via the hypogastric nerve
- Relaxation of the detrusor muscle (β_3-adrenoceptors)
- The end result is detrusor inhibition and outlet excitation, leading to continent storage.

During rest, pelvic floor musculature and urethral properties also contribute to continence. As mentioned previously, urethral coaptation results from the integrity of the mucosa and submucosa. In addition, slow-twitch muscle fibres in the paraurethral layer of the external sphincter maintain passive continence by tonic contraction of the urethra.

The mechanism undergoes several adaptations during periods of increased intra-abdominal pressure.

- First, a reflex contraction of the levator ani musculature and urogenital diaphragm elevates suburethral supporting tissue and compresses the proximal urethra ('hammock hypothesis')

- Secondly, the urethropelvic ligaments envelop the proximal urethra and bladder neck medially and insert laterally onto the arcus tendineus fascia pelvis, augmenting the muscular closure of the pelvic floor
- Third, voluntary contraction of the fast-twitch fibres in the striated sphincter produces urethral compression.

In the setting of intact urethral support, increased intra-abdominal pressure is transmitted equally to the bladder and urethra, and the net effect is increased outlet resistance.

3.4 **Pathophysiology of overactive bladder syndrome**

OAB is often associated with DO, an urodynamic observation characterized by involuntary detrusor contractions during bladder filling. While symptoms such as urgency and UUI are sequelae of DO, many factors can influence its development:

- Hormonal changes, bladder outlet obstruction (BOO), ageing, ischaemia, and concomitant neurological and non-neurological conditions have been cited as factors potentially affecting bladder function
- Mechanisms contributing to OAB symptoms may be sensory or motor, and may be neurogenic, myogenic, mixed, or idiopathic in origin
- Additionally, various receptors and neurotransmitters associated with the urothelium may have a role in generating OAB symptoms.

Traditionally, DO was thought to result from a decreased capacity to handle increased afferent information or from a loss or decrease of the tonic inhibition of afferent impulses. During normal bladder filling, suprapontine inhibition can be voluntarily increased in response to bladder contractions. However, suprapontine inhibition may be affected in conditions such as stroke. Subsequently, involuntary detrusor contractions may be generated from low intensity afferent input and at lower bladder volumes.

The 'myogenic theory' proposes that morphological changes in the detrusor may be associated with OAB. Progressive denervation and hypertrophy of the bladder wall may be seen after BOO, neurogenic insult, and even normal ageing. Non-detrusor components and extracellular matrix composition may also be altered in these conditions. The resulting 'patchy denervation' of the detrusor may lead to increased excitability between detrusor myocytes and areas of denervation may correspond to individual muscle 'modules' that develop an increased sensitivity to neurotransmitters such as Ach. This increased muscular excitability leads to increased ability for activity to spread among cells and, subsequently, local uncoordinated detrusor contractions can lead to an increase in afferent signalling. This pathway may serve as a link between the neurogenic and myogenic theories of OAB.

Recently, a cascade of further peripheral events that may result in DO has been proposed:

• An enhanced reaction to heightened wall tension and stretching of the detrusor smooth muscle leads to increased afferent signalling during bladder filling

• Additional increased afferent activity may result from increased urothelial signalling to suburothelial nerves (as may be seen in BOO and normal ageing)

• This may be due to an increased amount of Ach released from the urothelium during bladder filling, above and beyond the typical basal Ach release

• The increase in Ach release from neuronal and non-neuronal (urothelial) sources increases the sensitivity of the detrusor to neurotransmitters and the resultant micromotion of the detrusor increases the afferent signalling in the suburothelium and detrusor. This leads to the sensation of urgency.

Changes in intracellular communication between myocytes seen with BOO may also contribute to symptoms of OAB. As detrusor cells are believed to be electrically coupled, gap junctions are believed to be abnormal in bladders of patients with DO. Thus, increases in receptor-mediated muscle contractility and interaction between smooth muscles cells may result in coordinated myogenic contraction of the entire bladder and DO.

3.5 Pathophysiology of stress urinary incontinence

SUI is thought to result from a deficiency in intrinsic, extrinsic, or combined support.

A defect in the mucosal seal may result in SUI:

• The urethra may be simultaneously subjected to both expulsive and shearing forces during stress manoeuvres and incontinence results when the sum of these forces overcomes urethral coaptation and disrupt the urethral seal

• Decreased arterial inflow to the mucosal layer secondary to oestrogen deficiency, radiation, or prior surgery, may lower intraurethral pressure and contribute to SUI.

Damage to the external support may also result in SUI:

- Damage to the para-urethral or peri-urethral layer of the striated sphincter and the pelvic muscles or fasciae may affect tonic contraction and dynamic contraction during stress manoeuvres
- In women with loss of anatomic support, the proximal urethra descends during stress manoeuvres and rotates out of the pelvis
- Additionally, the bladder receives greater intra-abdominal pressure relative to the urethra. This may result in posterior urethral wall descent, bladder neck funnelling, and unexpected bladder neck opening
- Previous delivery, obesity, alterations in pudendal nerve function, and pelvic surgery are some of the risk factors for compromising effective urethral compression
- Furthermore, retroperitoneal surgery, disk disease, or myelodysplasia may lead to tonic incompetence of the bladder neck from damage to α-1 fibres originating in the thoracolumbar spinal cord and travelling in the hypogastric nerve.

Leakage of urine into the proximal urethra during stress manoeuvres may produce a urethra-to-bladder reflex, wherein stimulation of afferent axons in the pudendal nerve can initiate or increase DO. This theory may connect SUI and UUI.

The mid-urethra has also been postulated to be the site of maximal intraurethral pressure and implicated in SUI. Three opposing muscle forces have been identified that influence the micturition mechanism:

- A forward force activated by the pubococcygeous muscle
- A backward force activated by the levator ani musculature
- An inferior force controlled by the longitudinal muscle of the anus.

During an increase in intra-abdominal pressure, contraction of the pubococcygeous pulls the anterior vaginal wall forward and closes off the urethra, a response contingent on an intact attachment between the anterior vaginal wall and the pubo-urethral ligaments (PUL). Laxity in the PUL contributes to urethral funnelling and incontinence during stress manoeuvres.

Key references

Abrams P, Andersson KE, Birder L, et al. (2010). Fourth International Consultation on Incontinence recommendation of the International Scientific Committee: evaluation and treatment of urinary incontinence, pelvic organ prolapse, and faecal incontinence. *Neurourol Urodyn*, **29**, 213–40.

Andersson KE (2003). Storage and voiding symptoms: pathophysiologic aspects. *Urology*, **62**, 3–10.

Andersson KE (2004). Antimuscarinics for treatment of overactive bladder. *Lancet Neurol*, **3,** 46–53.

DeLancey JO (1994). Structural support of the urethra as it relates to stress urinary incontinence: the hammock hypothesis. *Am J Obstet Gynecol*, **170**, 1713–23.

Ouslander JG (2004). Management of overactive bladder. *N Engl J Med*, **350**, 786–99.

Petros PE, Ulmsten U (1990). An integral theory of female urinary incontinence. *Acta Obstet Gynecol Scand*, **69**, 7–31.

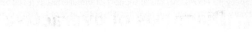

Chapter 4

Diagnosis of overactive bladder syndrome and stress urinary incontinence

Alexander Gomelsky & Roger R. Dmochowski

Key points

- A comprehensive history and physical examination is the keystone of diagnosing urinary incontinence and lower urinary tract symptoms.
- Urinalysis should be considered an extension of the physical examination and should be performed in every patient.
- Non-invasive uroflow may provide valuable information regarding the voiding phase; however, this study is insufficient to diagnose bladder outlet obstruction.
- Filling cystometry with valsalva leak point pressure determination may help guide therapeutic decisions in patients with stress urinary incontinence.

4.1 Introduction

The fourth International Consultation on Incontinence has recently released its recommendations regarding the nomenclature, diagnosis, and treatment of urinary incontinence. Each of the 23 committees has written a report on the published scientific work in order to give evidence-based recommendations.

- A highly recommended test should be done in every patient
- A recommended test is a test of proven value in the evaluation of most patients and its use is strongly encouraged during initial evaluation
- An optional test is a test of proven value in the evaluation of selected patients and its use is left to the clinical judgment of the physician.

4.2 **Highly recommended tests during initial evaluation**

4.2.1 **History**

The history is important in assessing the characteristics and severity of the incontinence, as well as its impact on quality of life (QoL). In absence of other diagnostic modalities, a detailed history may often provide sufficient information to make a proper diagnosis.

History of present illness

Symptom characteristics:

- Character and precipitating factors (urgency vs. stress manoeuvres) or is leakage continuous or insensate?
- Frequency of episodes (transient vs. daily)
- Onset and duration (acute vs. long-term)
- Timing (daytime, night-time, or diurnal)
- Exacerbating and alleviating factors
- Type and timing of fluid intake
- Associated symptoms: urgency, frequency, nocturia, dysuria, haematuria, pelvic pain, dyspareunia, difficulty emptying bladder
- Use of pads, diapers, or other protective devices
- Impact on QoL (What activities are affected by incontinence? Does urinary leakage contribute to depression?)
- Previous conservative, medical, and surgical treatments, as well as their effectiveness and side effects
- Any leakage during intercourse in women at penetration (more representative of stress urinary incontinence) or orgasm (more representative of overactive bladder syndrome)
- Goals and expectations of treatment should be assessed.

Past medical history

- Gravity, parity; types of deliveries; menopausal status; hormone replacement history
- Hypertension, diabetes, coronary artery disease, Alzheimer's disease
- Neurological conditions: stroke, multiple sclerosis, spinal cord injury, myelodysplasia, Parkinson's disease
- Abdominal and pelvic trauma
- Cancer of the cervix/uterus, bladder, and prostate
- Radiation therapy.

Past surgical history

- Pelvic, vaginal, urethral, and prostate surgery (including cystoscopy)

- Surgery for disc disease and orthopaedic surgery on lower extremities may indicate impaired mobility
- Previous craniotomy.

Medications

- Antimuscarinic medications for overactive bladder (OAB) syndrome, including previous use
- Alpha-adrenergic blockers for known or presumed benign prostatic obstruction
- Medicines, such as diuretics, for hypertension, diabetes, coronary artery disease, depression, Alzheimer's disease, and Parkinson's disease may impact urinary incontinence.

Social history

- History of tobacco use in the face of gross or microscopic haematuria may warrant an evaluation for bladder cancer. Alcohol consumption and the use of recreational drugs including ketamine can cause urinary symptoms
- Exercise regimen (if any)
- Support system, including living facility and caretakers
- Assessment of independence with activities of daily living.

Review of systems

- Effect of any symptoms on sexual and bowel function
- Assess recent weight gain or loss, vision changes, lower extremity oedema, back pain, paraesthesias, depression, and anxiety.

4.2.2 **Physical examination**

General considerations

General assessment includes an evaluation of mental status, obesity, physical dexterity and mobility. Impairment in orientation, cognition, and understanding may impact the ability to implement the subsequent treatment plan.

Abdominal and flank examination

- Flank fullness or tenderness may indicate renal mass, infection, or infrarenal obstruction
- Abdominal masses may include hernias, ovarian or uterine pathology, or a distended bladder.

Female pelvic examination

- Perineum and external genitalia should be examined for excoriation or erythema
- Vaginal lining with thin and pale epithelium and with loss of rugae suggests urogenital atrophy
- Vaginal examination is ideally performed with a full bladder to evaluate incontinence and again with an empty bladder

- In lithotomy position, with a comfortably-full bladder, the patient is asked to cough and valsalva to reproduce stress urinary incontinence (SUI)
- Urethral mobility may be estimated by observation or with a well-lubricated, urethral cotton swab placed at the bladder neck. Urethral hypermobility is defined as a resting or straining angle greater than 30 degrees from the horizontal
- Evaluation of the anterior, posterior, and apical compartments is best performed while reducing the other compartments with a single-blade speculum
- Prolapse in each compartment may be graded using either the Baden-Walker (modified halfway; 0–4) grading system or more precisely using the pelvic organ prolapse quantification system (POP-Q)
- Anterior compartment prolapse should be reduced while cough and valsalva manoeuvres are performed to evaluate for occult SUI
- Asking the patient to contract their pelvic muscles during a vaginal examination may estimate pelvic muscle strength and may provide useful information regarding pelvic floor physiotherapy as a potential option for symptom treatment
- Rectal examination may further delineate the degree of rectocoele or perineal body weakness
- If incontinence is not reproduced in the lithotomy position, cough and valsalva manoeuvres may be repeated with the patient in the standing position and one foot on a stool.

Male examination

- The urethral meatus is examined for stenosis or hypospadias and foreskin for phimosis
- The penis, scrotum, testes, epididymides, and perineum should be examined
- Digital rectal examination (DRE) provides an estimate of prostate size, consistency, and symmetry
- In men who complain of incontinence following open or transurethral prostate surgery, incontinence should be assessed with cough and valsalva manoeuvres in the standing position.

Neurological examination

- A lax anal sphincter on DRE suggests possible neurologic damage
- The bulbocavernosus reflex is checked by squeezing the glans or clitoris and feeling the anal sphincter and perineal muscles contract
- Alternatively, an indwelling urethral catheter may be pulled to elicit anal and perineal muscle contraction

- The absence of this reflex in men is almost always associated with a neurological lesion, but the reflex may not be detectable in many neurologically intact women.

4.2.3 **Dipstick urinalysis should be performed in each patient**

The urinalysis screens for haematuria, glucosuria, proteinuria, pyuria, the presence of leucocyte esterase, and nitrite. Abnormal findings should be confirmed by microscopic evaluation of the urinary sediment. Confirmed abnormalities may prompt additional work-up for urologic cancer, stone disease, or infection. The finding of glucosuria may prompt a work-up for diabetes. Significant proteinuria may indicate underlying renal disease, while specific gravity may be a surrogate measurement for hydration status.

4.3 **Complementary investigations**

The following investigations are recommended prior to or during specialist assessment.

4.3.1 **Post-void residual determination**

If the patient is suspected of having voiding dysfunction, post-void residual determination (PVR) should be part of the initial assessment. PVR may be checked with urethral catheterization or by using a bladder ultrasound (least invasive method). In a single patient, PVR may vary and more than one measurement may be necessary. A non-representative PVR is common when the patient's bladder is not sufficiently full to yield a normal desire to void. A PVR alone should be interpreted cautiously, and should be used as a supporting piece of data in evaluating the patient.

4.3.2 **Flowmetry (uroflow)**

Uroflow represents the plotting of urine flow 'Q' (in cm^3 or mL) vs. time (in seconds). Urine flow is described in terms of rate (cm^3/sec) and pattern. The pattern may be intermittent or continuous. Amount voided is important, and uroflow volumes lower than 150 cm^3 should be interpreted with caution. A normal uroflow in a female is shown in Figure 4.1. Urine flow rate is a composite measure of the detrusor contraction and urethral resistance. Thus, a low uroflow may represent either bladder outlet obstruction (BOO), detrusor underactivity, or both. Uroflow may be especially useful in men (due to the high likelihood for BOO) and in women at risk for BOO (e.g. high-grade POP or previous anti-incontinence or anti-prolapse surgery), and those with an elevated PVR.

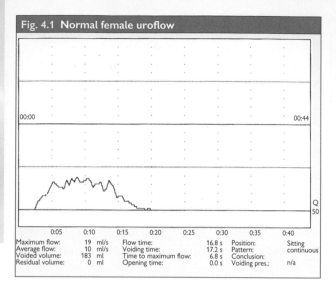

Fig. 4.1 Normal female uroflow

Maximum flow:	19 ml/s	Flow time:	16.8 s	Position:	Sitting
Average flow:	10 ml/s	Voiding time:	17.2 s	Pattern:	continuous
Voided volume:	183 ml	Time to maximum flow:	6.8 s	Conclusion:	
Residual volume:	0 ml	Opening time:	0.0 s	Voiding pres.:	n/a

4.4 Other investigations

4.4.1 Frequency-volume chart

The frequency-volume chart (FVC) gives the physician a representative measurement of fluid intake, voiding times and volumes, and circumstances leading to urinary incontinence. While the optimum number of days to record a FVC is controversial, a 3-day FVC appears to provide a good balance between diagnostic accuracy and patient compliance. For optimal effectiveness, all voids and incontinence episodes should be recorded. A FVC has also been found to be an excellent learning tool for patients to evaluate factors associated with their urinary incontinence. Additional criteria may be included on the FVC. These include:

- Degree of leakage (drops, teaspoons, emptied bladder contents)
- Number of pads or absorbent products used.

A sample FVC is found in Table 4.1.

4.4.2 Quality of Life questionnaires

It has been acknowledged that symptoms alone are poor indicators of the effect that incontinence has on a patient's life. Since the extent of the impact of incontinence to cause embarrassment and social disruption varies, measurement should provide self-reported (subjective) symptoms and their perceived impact; the International

Table 4.1 Sample frequency–volume chart					
Time	Amount voided (cm³)	# of leakage episodes	Activity during leak	Urgency with leak? (Y/N)	Fluid intake (mL/oz, type)
Midnight–3 a.m.					
3–6 a.m.					
6–9 a.m.					
9 a.m.–noon					
Noon–3 p.m.					
3–6 p.m.					
6–9 p.m.					
9 p.m.–midnight					

Consultation on Incontinence (ICI) has recommended the use of the validated ICI Questionnaire (ICIQ) modules (http://www.iciq.net). The recommended questionnaires for urinary incontinence, lower urinary tract symptoms, and overactive bladder are listed in Table 4.2 and Table 4.3. The use of a particular questionnaire should be tailored toward the specific symptoms and patient. Outcomes may be followed longitudinally to gauge improvement or deterioration of symptoms.

4.4.3 Cystometry

Definition

Filling cystometry is the method by which changes in bladder pressure are measured during bladder filling (Figure 4.2). This study requires urethral catheterization, and typically a second catheter (placed vaginally or rectally) to simultaneously measure abdominal pressures. The patient should be upright, or in the sitting position for the study. The bladder is filled with liquid, usually at 50 mL/min, and several values are recorded during filling cystometry.

The following values indicating bladder sensation are noted:

- Volume at first desire to void
- Volume at normal desire to void
- Volume at strong desire to void
- Volume at urgency

Table 4.2 International Consultation on Incontinence Questionnaire (ICIQ) Modular Structure (http://www.iciq.net)

Condition	Recommended modules	Optional modules	QoL	Generic QoL	Sexual matters	Post-treatment
	(A) Core modules			Recommended add-on modules		
Urinary symptoms	Males: ICIQ-MLUTS Females: ICIQ-FLUTS	Males: ICIQ-MLUTS long form Females: ICIQ-FLUTS long form	ICIQ-LUTSqol	SF-12	Males: ICIQ-MLUTSsex Female: ICIQ-FLUTSsex	ICIQ-S (satisfaction)
Urinary incontinence	ICIQ-UI short form	ICIQ-UI long form	ICIQ-LUTSqol ICIQ-UIqol (optional)	SF-12	Males: ICIQ-MLUTSsex Female: ICIQ-FLUTSsex	
Condition	(B) Specific patient groups		QoL	Generic QoL	Sexual matters	
Nocturia	ICIQ-N		ICIQ-Nqol	SF-12	Males: ICIQ-MLUTSsex Female: ICIQ-FLUTSsex	
Overactive bladder	ICIQ-OAB		ICIQ-OABqol	SF-12	Males: ICIQ-MLUTSsex Female: ICIQ-FLUTSsex	

ICIQ-MLUTS, ICIQ-male lower urinary tract symptoms.
ICIQ-FLUTS: ICIQ-female lower urinary tract symptoms. ICIQ-MLUTS long form: ICIQ-male lower urinary tract symptoms long form.
ICIQ-FLUTS long form: ICIQ-female lower urinary tract symptoms long form.
ICIQ-UI short form: ICIQ-urinary incontinence form.
ICIQ-LUTSqol: ICIQ-lower urinary tract symptoms quality of life.
ICIQ-UIqol: ICIQ-urinary incontinence symptoms quality of life.

ICIQ-MLUTSsex: ICIQ-male sexual matters associated with lower urinary tract symptoms.
ICIQ-FLUTSsex: ICIQ-female sexual matters associated with lower urinary tract symptoms.
ICIQ-N: ICIQ-nocturia.
ICIQ-Nqol: ICIQ-nocturia quality of life.
ICIQ-OAB: ICIQ-overactive bladder.
ICIQ-OABqol: ICIQ-overactive bladder symptoms quality of life.

Table 4.3 Recommended questionnaires for urinary incontinence, lower urinary tract symptoms, and overactive bladder

Combined symptoms and QoL impact of urinary incontinence

Women	ICIQ-FLUTS
	BFLUTS-SF
	SUIQQ
Men	ICIQ-MLUTS
	ICSmale

Combined symptoms and QoL of overactive bladder

Men & Women	OAB-q, ICIQ-OAB

Urinary incontinence symptoms

Men & Women	ICIQ-UI SF
Women	UDI; UDI-6
	Incontinence severity index
	BFLUTS
Men	ICSmale
	Danish Prostatic Symptom Score

Quality of life impact of urinary incontinence

Men & Women	I-QOL
	SEAPI-QMM
	ICIQ-LUTSqol
Women	KHQ
	IIQ, IIQ-7
	UISS
	CONTILIFE
Men	None

ICIQ: International Consultation on Incontinence Questionnaire; MLUTS: Male Lower Urinary Tract Symptoms; FLUTS: Female Lower Urinary Tract Symptoms; UI SF: Urinary incontinence Short FormBFLUTS-SF: short form of the Bristol Female LUTS Questionnaire; SUIQQ: Stress and urge incontinence and quality of life questionnaire; ICSmale: International Continence Society Male; OAB-q: overactive bladder questionnaire; UDI: urogenital distress inventory; I-QOL: Quality of life in persons with urinary incontinence questionnaire; SEAPI-QMM: Incontinence classification system; KHQ: King's Health Questionnaire; IIQ: Incontinence impact questionnaire; UISS: urinary incontinence severity score; CONTILIFE: Quality of life assessment questionnaire concerning urinary incontinence.

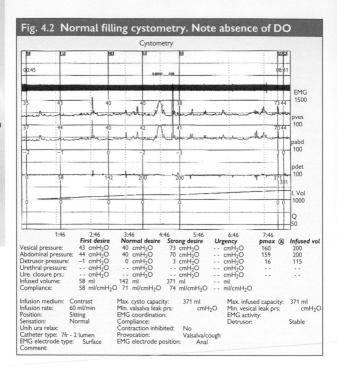

Fig. 4.2 Normal filling cystometry. Note absence of DO

	First desire	Normal desire	Strong desire	Urgency	pmax @	Infused vol
	2:46	3:46	4:46	5:46	6:46	7:46
Vesical pressure:	43 cmH₂O	40 cmH₂O	73 cmH₂O	-- cmH₂O	160	200
Abdominal pressure:	44 cmH₂O	40 cmH₂O	70 cmH₂O	-- cmH₂O	159	200
Detrusor pressure:	−1 cmH₂O	0 cmH₂O	3 cmH₂O	-- cmH₂O	16	115
Urethral pressure:	-- cmH₂O	-- cmH₂O	-- cmH₂O	-- cmH₂O	--	--
Ure. closure prs.:	-- cmH₂O	-- cmH₂O	-- cmH₂O	-- cmH₂O	--	--
Infused volume:	58 ml	142 ml	371 ml	-- ml		
Compliance:	58 ml/cmH₂O	71 ml/cmH₂O	74 ml/cmH₂O	-- ml/cmH₂O		

Infusion medium:	Contrast	Max. cysto capacity:	371 ml	Max. infused capacity:	371 ml
Infusion rate:	60 ml/min	Min. valsalva leak prs:	cmH₂O	Min. vesical leak prs:	cmH₂O
Position:	Sitting	EMG coordination:		EMG activity:	
Sensation:	Normal	Compliance:		Detrusor:	Stable
Unih ura relax:		Contraction inhibited:	No		
Catheter type:	7fr - 2 lumen	Provocation:	Valsalva/cough		
EMG electrode type:	Surface	EMG electrode position:	Anal		
Comment:					

- Bladder sensation may be affected by the rate of bladder filling and temperature of the filling medium
- Conditions such as cystitis and OAB may often be accompanied by early sensations of bladder fullness, while conditions such as diabetes may be associated with delayed sensations.
- Maximum cystometric bladder capacity (in cm³): like bladder sensation, bladder capacity may be affected by rate of filling and temperature of filling medium.
- Compliance (change in volume divided by change in pressure)
  - innate physical properties of a healthy bladder wall allow for a low increase in intravesical pressure during bladder filling
  - a normal compliance is high (large change in volume divided by a minimal change in pressure)
  - compliance can be influenced by filling rate, patient position, and volume of fluid infused
  - decreased compliance can be found in myelodysplasia, radiation cystitis, and denervation following radical pelvic surgery

- Presence or absence of involuntary detrusor contractions (detrusor overactivity; DO):
  - previously, a phasic rise in detrusor pressure >15 cmH$_2$O was considered a threshold value for diagnosing DO; however, any degree of DO is currently considered significant when an involuntary rise in detrusor pressure reproduces the patient's symptoms
  - it is important to note that involuntary detrusor contractions in the absence of urgency are common and may be present in over two-thirds of normal, healthy women
  - the finding of DO coinciding with a feeling of urgency indicates that neural pathways in the pelvis and spinal cord are intact
  - a successful voluntary pelvic floor contraction that suppresses DO may indicate that pelvic floor physiotherapy may have a role in the treatment of the patient's symptoms.
- Valsalva leak point pressure (VLPP) or abdominal leak point pressure (Figure 4.3):
  - this is an indirect measure of the urethra's ability to withstand urinary leakage after an increase in abdominal pressure

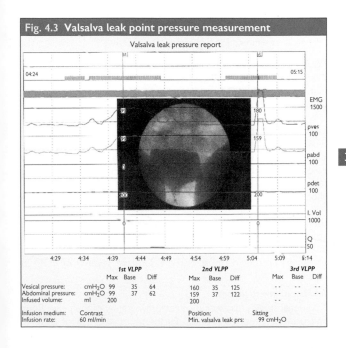

Fig. 4.3 Valsalva leak point pressure measurement

Valsalva leak pressure report

		1st VLPP			2nd VLPP			3rd VLPP	
		Max	Base	Diff	Max	Base	Diff	Max	Base	Diff
Vesical pressure:	cmH$_2$O	99	35	64	160	35	125	- -	- -	- -
Abdominal pressure:	cmH$_2$O	99	37	62	159	37	122	- -	- -	- -
Infused volume:	ml	200			200			- -		

Infusion medium:	Contrast	Position:	Sitting
Infusion rate:	60 ml/min	Min. valsalva leak prs:	99 cmH$_2$O

- to evaluate the VLPP, the patient is asked to cough and/or perform a valsalva manoeuvre several times during the filling cycle. The initial attempt is at 150–200 cm³ and then every 100–200 cm³ thereafter. The pressure at which leakage occurs is termed the VLPP
- traditionally, women with higher VLPP (>90 cmH$_2$O) were felt to have greater degrees of sphincter function, while women with VLPP <60 cmH$_2$O were considered to have intrinsic sphincter deficiency
- many surgeons have often based their decision to pursue a particular mode of therapy based on the VLPP.
- Detrusor leak point pressure (DLPP):
  - DLPP is a measure of the urethra's ability to withstand leakage during DO
  - classically, DLPP is an important measurement in patients with neurogenic bladder dysfunction, and specifically those with low compliance and urinary incontinence
  - if the DLPP is >40 cmH$_2$O at the time of leakage, then the patient is felt to be at risk for upper tract deterioration
  - patients with DLPP<40 cmH$_2$O, or those that can be pharmacologically or surgically manipulated to store at a pressure <40 cmH$_2$O, do not experience upper tract deterioration in the absence of infection or vesicoureteral reflux.

Voiding cystometry (pressure-flow study)

Pressure-flow study (PFS) is typically performed following filling cystometry, once bladder capacity has been reached and the patient initiates a voluntary void.

Intravesical pressure, intra-abdominal pressure (rectal or vaginal catheter), and uroflow are measured simultaneously. Urodynamically, BOO may be defined by the interaction between detrusor pressure during voiding and urinary flow rate. The normal adult male typically voids with a detrusor pressure of 40–60 cmH$_2$O, while the adult female voids with much lower pressures. As women have much shorter urethras, and therefore less outlet resistance, they may void with almost no rise in detrusor pressure. A high pressure void in the setting of low urinary flow indicates BOO in males; however, strict criteria to diagnose BOO in women are controversial. The International Continence Society (ICS) pressure-flow nomogram should be used to diagnose and measure the severity of BOO in males.

Additional Investigations

Additional studies may include electromyography of the pelvic floor and urethral pressure profiles. Furthermore, the use of isotonic contrast as a filling medium and simultaneous fluoroscopy may be extremely useful in diagnosing the aetiology of complex urinary incontinence.

Key references

Abrams P, Andersson KE, Birder L, Brubaker L, Cardozo L, Chapple C, *et al.* (2010). Fourth International Consultation on Incontinence recommendation of the International Scientific Committee: evaluation and treatment of urinary incontinence, pelvic organ prolapse, and faecal incontinence. *Neurourol Urodyn*, **29**, 213–240.

Avery KN, Bosch JL, Gotoh M, Naughton M, Jackson S, Radley SC, *et al.* (2007). Questionnaires to assess urinary and anal incontinence: review and recommendations. *J Urol,* **177**, 39–49.

Rovner ES, Wein AJ (2002). Practical urodynamics. *AUA Update Series,* Volume XXI, Lesson 19.

Rovner ES, Wein AJ (2002). Practical urodynamics. *AUA Update Series,* Volume XXI, Lesson 20.

Chapter 5

Treatment of overactive bladder syndrome and stress urinary incontinence

Hashim Hashim & Paul Abrams

> ## Key points
>
> - Treatment of overactive bladder (OAB) syndrome and stress urinary incontinence (SUI) can be divided into conservative, medical, and surgical treatments
> - Conservative treatments include patient and carer education, risk factor modification, bladder training, and pelvic floor muscle training
> - Antimuscarinics form the mainstay of medical treatment in OAB
> - There are no recognized medical treatments for SUI, however selective serotonin re-uptake inhibitors have been licensed in some countries for women with SUI
> - Surgical treatment of OAB includes intra-detrusor botulinum toxin injections, sacral nerve stimulation, bladder augmentation, detrusor myectomy or urinary diversion
> - Surgical treatment of SUI includes urethral bulking agents, mid-urethral synthetic slings, autologous slings, or artificial urinary sphincters.

5.1 Treatment of overactive bladder

Once patient assessment is complete, the health-care provider can initiate treatment. In almost all OAB groups no curative treatment can be offered, and this has to be explained to the patient and carers. The principles of treatment are to decrease urgency and thereby to reduce UUI episodes, frequency, nocturia, and to increase voided volume. Treatments include:

- Lifestyle interventions
- Bladder training and pelvic floor muscle training (PFMT)
- Pharmacotherapy
- Surgery
- Anti-incontinence devices.

The first three can be initiated in primary care. If they fail, then a specialist opinion should be sought (see Appendix).

5.1.1 **Lifestyle interventions**

Lifestyle interventions should include:

- Patient and carer education about the condition
- General and lifestyle measures such as reducing/stopping caffeine (which acts a mild diuretic and stimulant to the detrusor muscle) and alcohol intake
- Weight reduction which can help in mixed UI
- Stopping smoking, which helps reduce coughing and potentially cough-induced detrusor overactivity
- Advice on:
  - quantity, timing and type of fluid intake
  - quantity, timing of water-containing food intake
  - advice for specific occasions e.g. going shopping or to the cinema
  - empty bladder before going out or going to bed
  - empty bladder before intercourse
  - not drinking after 6 o'clock in the evening and voiding before going to bed, if nocturia is a problem
  - reducing fluid intake by 25% from normal as long as the patients are drinking more than 1 L of fluid per day. It is also important to remind patients that about 300–500 mL of fluid comes from water-containing foods such as fruits, vegetables and salads.

It is important to realize that, except for fluid reduction by 25%, none of the other treatments have strong an evidence-base to them. However, they are logical treatments that are cheap, easy to do, have no side effects and do work for some patients. It is therefore worth trying them, especially as OAB is a lifelong condition that may require several treatments.

5.1.2 **Bladder training and pelvic floor muscle training**

Bladder training aims to regain bladder control by suppressing involuntary detrusor contractions through increased feedback inhibition, thereby increasing the voided volumes and the time interval between voids, and improving the voiding pattern by reducing frequency. Bladder training consists of a scheduled toileting regimen whereby patients are taught to void regularly every hour on the hour whether they feel like voiding or not. If they normally void every 30 minutes then they should start with that rather than every hour. Once they have mastered the time frame between voids, they are asked to increase the duration between voids by 10 or 15 minutes each week until they feel comfortable with their urinary frequency. They should continue to do this for 3 or 4 months until they can control their voiding for at least 3 hours. Essentially, it is the brain controlling the bladder.

Bladder training is usually supplemented by pelvic floor muscle training (PFMT, Kegel exercises), where the patients are taught to tighten their pelvic floor when they get an involuntary contraction and when sitting-up from lying down and standing-up from a sitting position. These are both situations that can result in urgency and UUI due to an involuntary detrusor contraction. During bladder training and PFMT, the frequency/volume chart should be used to assess success and compliance in an objective manner.

These treatments are cheap and effective methods of reducing the symptoms of OAB, but it must be emphasized to the patient that they can take about 3 months to work and therefore they should persevere with the exercises and training.

There are many exercise instructions, which are available on the internet, such as http://www.continence-foundation.org.uk. One such regimen includes:

- Three sets of 8–12 slow velocity maximal voluntary pelvic floor muscle contractions
- Sustained for 6–8 seconds each
- Performed 3 or 4 times per week, and
- Continued for 15–20 weeks.

However, before asking the patients to do PFMT, the clinician must examine the patient to know that she or he can contract the pelvic floor. If the patient cannot, then referral to a specialist physiotherapist for consideration of electrotherapy is advised, with follow-up arranged after about 12 weeks.

Biofeedback and/or electrical stimulation can be used as adjuncts to bladder training in patients who are unable to locate or contract their pelvic floor muscles voluntarily by making subjects aware of normally unconscious physiological processes. However, in patients who can contract their pelvic floor, these adjuncts do not seem to provide any additive effect, in terms of efficacy, compared with bladder training alone.

Acupuncture has been used as an alternative treatment for OAB. Larger trials are needed to show whether the acupuncture is effective as it is safe, free of complications and side effects and may offer a therapy as effective as non-invasive treatments.

TENS (transcutaneous electrical nerve stimulation) is another non-invasive treatment, and involves placing surface electrodes on the skin. There is no consensus as to where to place the electrodes, how many treatments need to be given and how long each treatment should last. Sites that have been used include the thigh and abdomen. It is not known how TENS helps with OAB symptoms and it has not been subjected to double-blind controlled trials. There seems to be a subjective improvement, but no objective improvement when compared to oxybutynin. Further trials are required to assess its efficacy, especially in the long-term, and its cost-effectiveness. Nonetheless, it can be considered as a treatment option in patients, when symptoms are bothersome and conservative treatments have failed, but who do not want pharmacological or surgical treatment.

Up to 50% of patients may be content with conservative treatment if adhered to appropriately. They work for both men and women.

5.1.3 **Oral pharmacotherapy**

The main neurotransmitter at the nerve endings on the detrusor smooth muscle is acetylcholine (Ach), which acts on the M3-muscarinic receptors in the bladder. Ach is not only a transmitter in the bladder but also in many other organs. The situation is made more complex by the fact that there are five subtypes of muscarinic receptors (M1–M5) variously distributed throughout the body organs. Therefore, blocking the action of Ach can have effects all over the body.

In the detrusor, all five subtypes of muscarinic receptors have been demonstrated and although the predominant muscarinic receptor is M2, which accounts for two-thirds of the receptors, the M3-receptors that make up the other one-third, are the receptors that have been found to be predominantly responsible for the detrusor contraction. M3-receptors are also present in smooth muscle, salivary glands, the eyes, and brain. The ubiquity of M3 receptors explains why it has been difficult to develop bladder selective anticholinergic drugs, and why the side effects of constipation, dry mouth, blurred vision, and drowsiness are difficult to avoid. The other important receptors are M2-receptors, which are present in the heart, and their stimulation causes parasympathetically-induced bradycardia, and the M1-receptors found in the brain, which are said to facilitate memory. Therefore, blockage of the M2-receptor can lead to tachycardia and of the M1-receptor to memory loss.

Antimuscarinic drugs, which block the muscarinic Ach receptors, form the cornerstone and mainstay of medical pharmacological treatment for OAB, which, although effective, may be poorly tolerated with little long-term data on their use in clinical practice.

These drugs aim to reduce the symptoms of OAB due to DO, with out significantly depressing detrusor contraction during voiding, th resulting in clinical and quality of life improvements.

The best results in OAB are obtained by combining antimuscarinics with bladder training and other conservative treatments.

Currently there are seven main antimuscarinic anticholinergic drugs, namely: oxybutynin, tolterodine, propiverine, trospium, solifenacin, darifenacin, and fesoterodine. All these drugs were given Level 1 evidence and Grade A recommendation in the fourth International Consultation on Incontinence (ICI) for the treatment of OAB (Table 5.1).

Oxybutynin chloride

- First antimuscarinic used for the treatment of OAB
- Approved in 1972
- Tertiary amine with:
  - anticholinergic effects on smooth muscle, including the bladder
  - antispasmodic effects on the detrusor muscle.
- Short half-life with high affinity for the M1 and M3 muscarinic receptors of the bladder and parotid gland
- Undergoes extensive hepatic first-pass metabolism
- Active metabolite, N-desethyloxybutynin, has similar properties to the parent drug and thus contributes to oxybutynin's pharmacological effects
- Has musculotropic, smooth muscle-relaxant effects and local anaesthetic effects
- Onset of action is within 30–60 minutes of administration
- Peak effects occur within 3–6 hours of administration

Table 5.1 International Consultation on Urological Diseases (ICUD) guidelines for levels of evidence and grades of recommendation (modified from the Oxford Centre for Evidence-Based Medicine; http://www.cebm.net/index.aspx?o=1025)

Levels of evidence	Grades of recommendation
1 Systematic reviews, meta-analysis, good quality randomized controlled trials	**A** Based on Level 1 evidence (highly recommended)
2 Less good quality randomized-controlled trials, good quality prospective cohort studies	**B** Consistent Level 2 and 3 evidence (recommended)
3 Case-control studies, case series	**C** Level 3 studies or 'majority evidence' (optional)
4 Expert opinion	**D** Evidence inadequate and/or conflicting (no recommendation possible)

available in three main formulations:

- *oral tablet immediate-release*—available in doses of 2.5, 3, and 5 mg. Can be used up to three times daily with a maximum daily dose of 20 mg
- *oral tablet extended-release*—once daily 5 and 10mg tablet, maximum daily dose of 20 mg
- *topical transdermal patch*—one patch on the skin every 3 days; 36 mg/patch (3.9 mg/day); main side effect is pruritis and therefore site of application of the patch needs to be changed each time

- The rectal and intravesical routes have also been used in the administration of oxybutynin to avoid hepatic first-pass metabolism. These routes should only be used in patients who cannot tolerate the oral or transdermal routes or in whom other treatments have failed. Electromotive drug administration has also been used to deliver oxybutynin intravesically, but has not been a very popular method, possibly due to the high costs of the device and catheters
- Oxybutynin is the only antimuscarinic licensed in children.

Tolterodine tartrate

- Launched in 1998
- Synthetic tertiary amine
- Competitive non-selective muscarinic receptor antagonist
- *In vivo*, greater selectivity for the bladder over salivary glands
- Undergoes extensive first-pass metabolism in the liver
- Administered orally
- Two formulations:
  - *standard release form*—1 and 2 mg tablets, which can be administered twice daily; maximum dose is 4 mg/day; peak serum concentrations within 1–2 hours after administration
  - *extended-release form*—4mg tablets administered once a day; maximum dose is 4 mg/day; peak serum concentration 2–6 hours after administration
- Half-life:
  - 3 hours for extensive metabolizers
  - 10 hours for poor metabolizers
- Dose can be adjusted according to individual clinical response and tolerance.

Propiverine hydrochloride

- Tertiary amine
- Calcium-channel blocking action *in vitro*

- Undergoes extensive first-pass metabolism
- Three active metabolites
- Reaches peak plasma levels in about 2.5 hours
- Eliminated in urine, bile, and faeces
- Two oral formulations:
  - *immediate-release*—15mg tablets with maximum dose of three times per day (45 mg/day)
  - *modified-release*—30 mg tablets once a day with maximum dose of 30 mg/day.

Solifenacin succinate

- Selective M1 and M3 receptors antagonist in the bladder
- Primarily cleared by hepatic metabolism, but some urinary excretion
- Maximum concentrations reached after 3–8 hours
- Terminal half-life is 45–68 hours
- One pharmacologically active and three inactive metabolites
- *Oral tablet:* 5 and 10 mg once daily doses; maximum dose is 10 mg/day.

Darifenacin hydrobromide

- Selective muscarinic M3 receptor antagonist
- Extensively metabolized by the liver following oral administration
- Maximum plasma levels reached in about 7 hours
- Excreted in urine and faeces
- Elimination half-life is 13–19 hours
- *Oral tablet:* 7.5 and 15 mg once daily doses; maximum daily dose is 15 mg.

Fesoterodine fumarate

- Competitive, non-selective muscarinic receptor antagonist
- Rapidly and extensively hydrolysed by non-specific plasma esterases to the same active metabolite as tolterodine
- Maximum plasma levels reached after about 5 hours
- Terminal half-life of active metabolite is about 7 hours
- *Two oral doses:* 4 and 8 mg once a day; maximum daily dose is 8 mg.

Trospium chloride

- Quaternary amine
- Competitive inhibitor of Ach at muscarinic receptors with equal selectivity for the M3 and M2-receptors

- Has been used in Europe for more than 20 years and approved by the United States Food and Drug Administration (FDA) in 2004
- It is hydrophilic and therefore should not cross the blood brain barrier, as may the tertiary amines
- In theory, central nervous system and cognitive performance side effects such as dizziness should be minimal
- Reaches peak plasma concentration after 4–6 hours
- Poorly absorbed from the gastrointestinal tract—80% is excreted in the faeces as the active parent compound
- *Two oral formulations:*
  - *immediate-release*—20 mg tablets twice daily; maximum dose is 40 mg/day; terminal elimination half-life is 20 hours
  - *extended-release*—60 mg capsule once a day; maximum dose is 60 mg/day; terminal elimination half-life is 38.5 hours.

Side effects and contraindications of antimuscarinics

The main side effects include:

- Dry mouth
- Constipation
- Dizziness
- Dry eyes
- Headache.

The main contraindications include:

- Urinary retention
- Uncontrolled narrow angle glaucoma
- Myasthenia gravis
- Known hypersensitivity to excipients
- Severe ulcerative colitis
- Toxic megacolon.

Other pharmacological agents

Although antimuscarinics form the cornerstone of medical treatment for OAB, they are not without side effects. Also, the antimuscarinic receptor specificities observed *in vitro*, may not be translated into differing clinical efficacy between the drugs.

Other oral pharmacological agents have been used for the treatment of OAB. However, the level of evidence available is not sufficient for them to be used generally, although some physicians continue to use and prescribe them. These include:

- Oestrogens (Level 2, Grade C)
- Flavoxate (Level 2, Grade D)
- Imipramine (Level 3, Grade C)

- Propantheline (Level 2, Grade B)
- Tamsulosin (Level 3, Grade C)
- Terbutaline (Level 3, Grade C)
- Phosphodiesterase inhibitors (Level 2, Grade B)
- Prostaglandin synthesis inhibitors, such as flurbiprofen and indomethacin (Level 2, Grade C)
- Calcium antagonists, such as nifedipine and diltiazem (Level 2, Grade D)
- Serotonin norepinephrine re-uptake inhibitors (SNRIs), such as duloxetine (Level 2, Grade C)
- Potassium channel openers, such as pinacidil and cromokalim (Level 2, Grade D)—not available in the UK
- Gabapentin
- Desmopressin (Level 2, Grade C in OAB; Level 1, Grade A in nocturia).

Antimuscarinics and combination therapy

Patients who suffer with OAB can sometimes have other lower urinary tract symptoms (LUTS), such as stress urinary incontinence (SUI) or voiding symptoms. There are studies to suggest that the use of antimuscarinics with alpha-blockers in men with benign prostatic obstruction does not increase the risk of urinary retention in men with voiding LUTS.

There are no studies on the use of antimuscarinics for OAB seen in combination with desmopressin used for nocturia, or with duloxetine for stress UI, in patients who have mixed UI. However, since these drugs work by different mechanisms, it is possible to combine medications in order to treat conditions of different aetiologies. It is, however, important to warn patients that we do not have good evidence from trials, so cannot give strong support to such combinations.

Which oral agent to use?

When choosing an antimuscarinic drug the balance has to be between efficacy and side effects. When prescribing, enquiries about concomitant diseases should be made, in particular renal failure and hepatic failure as they can affect the metabolism and elimination of antimuscarinic drugs.

Physicians should be careful when prescribing antimuscarinics to elderly patients as the elimination time of the drug may be increased, for example, with oxybutynin, and because elderly patients are more likely to be taking other drugs, giving rise to potential drug interactions.

The decision to choose one drug over another is difficult and is probably governed by which drugs are licensed by national and local drug authorities, availability at the local hospital or in the community, and the cost of the drug, especially in countries where medications are not subsidized by the government.

The National Institute for Health and Clinical Excellence (NICE) in the UK recommends that oxybutynin immediate-release should be first-line treatment as there is no consistent evidence to suggest that one antimuscarinic is more efficacious than the other and since generic oxybutynin immediate-release is the cheapest one, it would be the most cost-effective. However, this recommendation was not popular with specialists as they felt it did not take into account the side effect profile of the different drug formulations and their tolerability. If oxybutynin immediate-release is used, patients should probably be reviewed in 2 weeks after starting the treatment to assess efficacy and tolerability, and if not tolerating the medication because of side effects then it should be changed to one of the other antimuscarinics. If the side effects are tolerated and more relief of symptoms is required, then the dose can be increased accordingly.

All the previous treatments can be initiated in primary care. When patients are referred to secondary care, it is our practice to try three different antimuscarinics before referring the patient for urodynamics to confirm detrusor overactivity and initiating more invasive treatments including intravesical therapy, neuromodulation or surgery.

5.1.4 **Intravesical pharmacotherapy**

Botulinum toxin A

Botulinum toxin A (BTA) selectively blocks the release of Ach from nerve endings and has been used by some urologists as second-line treatment for neurogenic DO, with good results (Level 2, Grade A). There are different formulations of BTA, but most studies have investigated onabotulinumtoxin (Botox® by Allergan).

Idiopathic DO is the most common type of DO, yet limited data are available on the use of BTA in this group of patients (Level 3 evidence, Grade B). It is still not licensed for this use although it has been used off-license.

BTA can be administered under local anaesthesia with a flexible cystoscope in the outpatient setting. Effects last about 6–9 months, after which the injections have to be repeated. Patients normally continue with antimuscarinics for 2 weeks after the procedure until the BTA takes full effect. They are given antibiotics for 5 days after the procedure to reduce the risk of urinary tract infections. Patients are taught intermittent self-catheterization (ISC) before performing the procedure as there is a 10–30% risk of urinary retention requiring ISC.

The long-term effects of using BTA are not known. Also, it is not established yet what the optimum dose of BTA to be used and at what sites to inject in the bladder and what the dose of each injection should be.

Resiniferatoxin

Resiniferatoxin (RTX), is an ultra-potent analogue of capsaicin and belongs to a group of substances known as vanilloids. These compounds act selectively on vanilloid subtype-1 receptors to desensitize unmyelinated afferent C-fibres. These fibres are responsible for detecting noxious stimuli and initiating painful sensations in the bladder of normal individuals. In neurogenic patients, the C-fibre afferents are activated and provide an additional afferent pathway in the micturition reflex.

These drugs seem to be used mainly in a clinical trial setting and have not gained popularity for use with the general public because of side effects. Also, RTX is not in clinical development due to formulation problems (Level 2, Grade C).

5.1.5 Neuromodulation

Sacral nerve stimulation (SNS) and percutaneous tibial nerve stimulation (PTNS) are new modalities that have been used in some centres world-wide and will probably help bridge the gap between pharmacotherapy and major surgery. There is more evidence from randomized control trials for SNS than there is for PTNS and, hence, SNS has been recommended for use by NICE in the UK for urgency incontinence.

The process of neuromodulation by SNS is not completely understood, but seems to involve modulation of spinal cord reflexes and brain networks by peripheral afferents, rather than direct stimulation of the motor response of the detrusor or urethral sphincter. In OAB, it seems to be successful in reducing frequency, UUI episodes and nocturia, as well as increasing bladder capacity and bladder volume at both first bladder sensation and normal desire to void. It also improves the quality of life of patients. The procedure can be done as a day case, under local or general anaesthesia, and involves two phases. Patients initially are implanted with a temporary lead in the test stimulation phase, which forms the primary nerve evaluation. If they have improvement in symptoms, which are objectively evaluated by a frequency/volume chart, the permanent tined lead and neurostimulator device are implanted into the S3 sacral nerve and buttock, respectively. The neurostimulator is operated by a battery that needs to be changed every 5–10 years. SNS is expensive, but it may be cheaper than surgery and its complications.

PTNS is less invasive than SNS, and has been approved by the FDA and European authorities. It involves inserting a needle electrode proximal to the medial malleolus above the ankle. This modulates the sacral nerve plexus via the peripheral nervous system by stimulating the afferent nerve fibres of the tibial nerve, and thus controls symptoms of OAB. The treatment is done in 30 minute sessions for 12 sessions and can be repeated as required.

5.1.6 **Surgery**

Surgery should be the last resort in the treatment of intractable OAB after failure of all the above treatments. Surgical options tried in the past included bladder distension, bladder transection, and transvaginal denervation. These techniques had short-term benefits, high recurrence rates and sometimes, high complication rates. Surgical rhizotomy is another procedure, but is limited to patients with spinal cord injuries because of its effects on the motor and sensory nerves.

The current existing surgical options aim to abolish urgency and UUI by increasing functional bladder capacity and thus reducing detrusor pressure at this capacity. These include augmentation cystoplasty, which aims to increase functional bladder capacity, detrusor myectomy, which removes part of the bladder smooth muscle, and finally urinary diversion when all else fails. These techniques seem to offer better results than the previous procedures but, like any operation, they have their own complications such as recurrent infections and bowel obstruction.

5.1.7 **Anti-incontinence and containment devices**

Anti-incontinence devices, such as urinary catheters, can be used as adjuncts to conservative and medical treatment or as an alternative to surgery in selected patients. They do, however, require knowledge of genital anatomy by the patients, and also the manual dexterity to insert and remove these devices. In addition to that, they may cause discomfort and have associated costs.

5.2 **Treatment of stress urinary incontinence**

Treatment of stress urinary incontinence can also be sub-classified similarly to that of OAB.

5.2.1 **Lifestyle interventions**

Lifestyle interventions regarding body weight, exercise, diet, and smoking, for the treatment of SUI, are often recommended by health-care professionals.

Weight loss is often recommended for women who have SUI, since obesity is an independent risk factor for SUI. However, there is only Level 2 evidence, but Grade A recommendation that weight loss in morbidly obese women decreases SUI and some Level 1 evidence that moderately obese women who lose weight have less SUI than those who do not.

Incontinence is often more exaggerated in some women while exercising and thus they may be advised not to exercise in order to stop the leakage if they choose not to have therapy for SUI. However, there is only Level 2/3 evidence to suggest that active women or those involved in heavy lifting are more likely to have SUI than those that do not. There are no trials looking at whether stopping exercise reduces SUI. On the contrary, exercising may play a role in strengthening the pelvic floor muscles and may be encouraged.

The effect of smoking on SUI is conflicting. It seems to increase the risk of severe SUI, but there are no data available as to whether stopping smoking reduces SUI. On the one hand, smokers are more likely to have violent coughing and therefore to increase their abdominal pressures causing SUI, while on the other hand they seem to have stronger urethral sphincters.

Other lifestyle interventions that have been tried include avoiding constipation since straining may be a risk factor for pelvic organ prolapse and SUI. Also crossing the legs and bending forwards may decrease SUI. However there are no trials available to suggest that reducing constipation or changing posture decreases SUI.

Trials in men are very scarce and no recommendations can be made, but it would seem logical to use the same advice given to women.

5.2.2 Pelvic floor muscle training

Pelvic floor muscle training (PFMT) involves voluntary contraction by tightening and squeezing the pelvic floor muscles to prevent leakage. Different mechanisms may be involved by which PFMT prevents SUI. A well-timed strong and fast pelvic floor contraction can prevent SUI by squeezing the urethra and increasing the intra-urethral pressure above the intra-abdominal pressure, as well as possibly preventing urethral descent and pushing the urethra against the back of the symphysis pubis.

Many different training programs have been proposed for PFMT (see Chapter 5), and are easily available on the world-wide-web or in print from continence foundations. They all seem to be better than placebo in the treatment of SUI, but it has to be remembered that an intensive and well supervised programme, within service constraints, provides better results than a simple unsupervised programme. Unfortunately, well supervised programmes are not available in all healthcare systems, and are mainly available in Northern European countries. Thus, providing written instructions to patients and regular follow-up with patient motivation is probably the next best thing and achieves good results in some patients.

Since PFMT are cheap, easy, and effective with no side effects, they should be used as first line therapy in the treatment of SUI in men and women. However, patients need persistence and dedication, as does the person treating them, since the therapeutic effects are not immediately apparent. It is advisable to use bladder diaries and QoL questionnaires, such as the International Consultation on Incontinence questionnaires (ICIQ; http://www.iciq.net), in the assessment of treatment effects in patients treated with PFMT.

In women, if there is no improvement in patient's perceived symptoms after 3 months of treatment, assuming patient compliance, then the patient should be re-evaluated and different treatment options considered.

In men, it is usually only seen post-prostatectomy. In such patients, PFMT should be continued for 6–12 months. PFMT can be taught pre-operatively and in the immediate post-operative period (Grade B). If no response is seen after 6 months then the patient, if troubled by his incontinence, should be referred for further treatment.

5.2.3 Oral pharmacotherapy

Pharmacological treatment of SUI aims to increase urethral closure pressure by increasing urethral smooth and striated muscle tone.

The basis for use of these drugs includes the presence of different types of receptors in the human bladder and urethra. The receptors in the bladder include $\beta1$, $\beta2$, and $\beta3$-adrenoceptors and muscarinic receptors while in the urethra the receptors include α- and β-adrenoceptors. Oestrogen receptors are present in both the bladder and urethra in women, and seem to play an important yet unidentified role in the continence mechanism. Serotonergic receptors, in Onuf's nucleus, also appear to play a role.

Oral pharmacological agents have been used mainly in women as very limited data is available in men.

Serotonin and norepinephrine reuptake inhibitors

Duloxetine hydrochloride is a balanced and potent dual reuptake inhibitor of serotonin and norepinephrine (NE). Both these neurotransmitters are believed to play key roles in lower urinary tract function. Serotonin suppresses parasympathetic activity and enhances sympathetic and somatic activity causing bladder relaxation and increasing outlet resistance, thus promoting urine storage. NE variably affects lower urinary tract function depending on the receptor subtype it interacts with. Serotonin and NE amplify the effect of glutamate on urethral striated muscle contraction. Glutamate is an excitatory neurotransmitter in bladder and urethral striated muscle reflex pathways and plays a role in initiating urethral striated muscle contraction during bladder filling. In the voiding phase there is suppression of glutamate transmission, which will result in inhibition of sphincter contraction and relaxation of the urethral striated muscle, and thus bladder emptying.

During bladder filling, duloxetine is thought to act centrally in the nervous system by stimulating sacral pudendal motor neurones via α_1-adrenergic and 5-hydroxytryptamine-2 ($5HT_2$) receptors by increasing the concentration of 5-HT and NE in Onuf's nucleus and thus amplifying the effect of glutamate. The increase in pudendal nerve activity increases striated urethral rhabdosphincter contractility and promotes urethral closure during filling.

This central mode of action through the sacral cord pudendal nerve nucleus implies that the cardiovascular class effect of α-adrenergics is reduced. In fact in the trials, duloxetine did not affect blood pressure significantly or cause changes in the electrocardiogram.

Nausea is the main side effect with duloxetine. It is generally well tolerated ranging from mild to moderate and lasting between 1 and 4 weeks. One way of reducing the risk of nausea is to start duloxetine treatment with 20 mg twice daily for 2 weeks, then increasing the dose to the recommended 40 mg twice daily. Other common adverse events observed in the clinical studies were dry mouth, fatigue, insomnia, constipation, headache, dizziness, somnolence, and diarrhoea.

Duloxetine (Level 1 evidence) is licensed at 40 mg twice daily for the treatment of SUI in the European Union, but not in the USA. Interestingly, it has also been licensed as an antidepressant at 60 mg once daily. There have been some reports by the FDA of increased suicidal ideation in adults with depression on antidepressants, but none have been reported in the clinical trials on incontinence since most were patients who did not have depression to start with.

In a randomized controlled trial of duloxetine alone, PFMT alone, combined treatment and no active treatment of women with SUI, it was found that combination therapy of duloxetine and PFMT was more efficacious in reducing urinary incontinence episodes than either alone.

Alpha-adrenoceptor (α-AR) agonists

α-AR agonists such as ephedrine, norephedrine (Level 3 evidence), midodrine (Level 2 evidence) and methoxamine (Level 2 evidence) have been used in the treatment of SUI. These drugs have been limited by their side effects of increasing blood pressure, headache, tremor, and sleep disturbances. Of these drugs, only midodrine has been licensed, and only in Finland, for the treatment of SUI.

Beta2-adrenoceptor (β_2-AR) agonists

β_2-AR agonists, such as clenbuterol, can increase urethral closure pressure by increasing the contractility of fast contracting striated muscle fibres through potentiation of Ach at the neuromuscular junction. It was initially developed as a bronchodilator. It has a Level 2 evidence for its effects, but has only been approved in Japan for treatment of SUI. Its side effects include tremor, headache, and tachycardia.

Tricyclic antidepressants

Imipramine is the main tricyclic antidepressant that has been used in incontinence. Its main use is in nocturnal enuresis in children, but has also been used in the treatment of SUI, UUI, and MUI. The mechanism of action of imipramine is not clear, but it does seem to have marked systemic anticholinergic action, as well as blockade of the reuptake of serotonin and norepinephrine. Imipramine also has cardiotoxic side effects including orthostatic hypotension and ventricular arrhythmias. There are no randomized controlled trials looking at the effects of imipramine in UUI, SUI, or MUI, but some open label studies have shown some beneficial effects in SUI (Level 3 evidence).

Oestrogens

Oestrogen is not objectively efficacious in the treatment of SUI when given alone. However when combined with other forms of therapy, such as other pharmacological agents or PFMT, then it may have a role.

5.2.4 **Surgery**

SUI is mainly caused by an anatomical defect and, hence, the main form of treatment, if PFMT fails, should be surgery to correct the anatomy as pharmacotherapy rarely works in SUI. Before embarking on a surgical treatment, urodynamics should be performed to confirm urodynamic stress incontinence (USI). There has been some debate as to whether urodynamics affects the outcome of surgery, and certainly, in the UK, NICE does not recommend performing urodynamics in cases of pure SUI diagnosed on history with no other LUTS. However, recent studies have shown that only 5–10% of women have pure stress incontinence symptoms.

Urethral bulking agents

Urethral bulking agents, such as collagen and silicon particles, have been used in men and women to treat SUI. They work by adding bulk and increase coaptation at the level of the bladder neck and external urethral sphincter. It can be done as a day case using a cystoscope. The main problems include the need for multiple injections, deterioration of effect over time, and very low cure rates.

In women cure rates range between 20 and 40%. In men, bulking therapy fails in up to 75% (Level 3; Grade C).

Abdominal surgery

Colposuspension has been the gold standard for the treatment of SUI in women. This has been largely superseded by mid-urethral synthetic slings. However, it still has a role in the treatment of recurrent SUI and in women who are having abdominal surgery such as a sacrocolpopexy. Laparoscopic colposuspension might be considered for the treatment of SUI in women who also require concurrent laparoscopic surgery for other reasons (Grade D), but should only be carried out by surgeons with specific training, expertise, and appropriate workload in laparoscopic incontinence surgery (Grade D).

Procedures such as the Marshall–Marchetti–Krantz (MMK), endoscopic or non-endoscopic needle suspension procedures, and paravaginal defect repairs are no longer recommended for SUI.

Slings

In women, synthetic and biological slings have been used. The main type of synthetic sling used is the mid-urethral retropubic transvaginal tape (TVT). A transobturator tape is also available. These are polypropelene meshes. We currently have 12-year data on TVTs. There are also adjustable and mini-slings being introduced into the market.

There is evidence that the retropubic TVT is as or more effective than the Burch colposuspension and equally effective as traditional fascial sling operations (Level 1/2). Operation time, hospital stay and time to resume normal daily activity is shorter with the TVT than with colposuspension. They are about 90% successful in terms of patient satisfaction rates. The main side effects are bladder perforation (5%) during surgery, post-operative urinary retention, tape erosion (4%) and exacerbation of other LUTS. The use of slings is not a contraindication in patients with OAB/detrusor overactivity, although women should be warned that OAB symptoms may persist after SUI surgery.

Autologous rectus fascial slings are the most widely used biological slings and are an effective treatment for SUI with proven longevity. However, the procedure does require more major surgery and, hence, has more side effects than synthetic slings.

In men, synthetic slings have recently become popular. There are no long-term data on their efficacy compared with the artificial urinary sphincter. However, they seem to be a reasonable alternative in men with lower and moderate degrees of incontinence, who have not had previous radiation, and have adequate detrusor contractility, or for patients demanding a less invasive procedure or non-mechanical device (Level 3; Grade C).

Artificial urinary sphincter

In men, the artificial urinary sphincter (AUS) is the gold standard treatment for SUI (Level 2; Grade B). On the other hand, in women, only Level 3/4 evidence, Grade B recommendation is available to support its use in SUI and it is mainly reserved for recurrent SUI.

In men, an adjustable balloon procedure has been used. Their use is based upon the concept of passive compression of the urethra utilising two balloons located on either side of the urethra. There are no long-term data to support its use and the replacement/revision may require multiple balloon re-fillings: there are also risks of urethral and bladder perforation.

5.3 **Treatment of mixed urinary incontinence**

Management of MUI should concentrate on a thorough history and examination to exclude other pathologies. Treatment expectations have to be realistic and strike a balance between patient's expectations and what is actually achievable and there should be a mutual decision between the patient and doctor as to how to proceed. Initial treatment concentrates on the most bothersome symptoms, and includes lifestyle interventions and pelvic floor muscle and bladder training. These can be combined with oral pharmacotherapy for optimum results.

Many different oral medications are available, however duloxetine is the only one used for stress-predominant MUI and antimuscarinics for the urgency-predominant MUI. Combining these two drug classes is also a feasible treatment option but, to date, this has not been subjected to a randomized controlled trial. If these treatment options fail, then further investigation is required with urodynamics to confirm the diagnosis. Once diagnosis is confirmed, there are invasive minor and major surgical procedures available for both components, SUI and UUI, but none have been evaluated in MUI. It has to be emphasized to patients that cure rates following surgery for SUI may be reduced and OAB symptoms will remain and may even worsen.

Assessment of patients with MUI should be continuous as some patients will feel better after conservative and medical treatment of their most predominant symptom and other symptoms may start to bother them and thus re-assessment is crucial.

Key references

Andersson KE, Chapple CR, Cardozo L, Cruz F, Hashim H, Michel MC, *et al.* (2009). Pharmacological treatment of overactive bladder: report from the International Consultation on Incontinence. *Curr Opin Urol,* **19**, 380–94.

Chapple CR, Khullar V, Gabriel Z, Muston D, Bitoun CE, Weinstein D (2008). The effects of antimuscarinic treatments in overactive bladder: an update of a systematic review and meta-analysis. *Eur Urol,* **54**, 543–62.

Dumoulin C, Hay-Smith J (2010). Pelvic floor muscle training versus no treatment, or inactive control treatments, for urinary incontinence in women. *Cochrane Database Syst Rev,* **1,** CD005654.

Hashim H, Al Mousa R (2009). Management of fluid intake in patients with overactive bladder. *Curr Urol Rep*, **10,** 428–33.

Herschorn S, Bruschini H, Comiter C, Grise P, Hanus T, Kirschner-Hermanns R, *et al.* (2010). Surgical treatment of stress incontinence in men. *Neurourol Urodyn*, **29,** 179–90.

Novara G, Artibani W, Barber MD, Chapple CR, Costantini E, Ficarra V, *et al.* (2010). Updated Systematic Review and Meta-Analysis of the Comparative Data on Colposuspensions, Pubovaginal Slings, and Midurethral Tapes in the Surgical Treatment of Female Stress Urinary Incontinence. *Eur Urol,* (Epub ahead of print).

Chapter 6

Treatment of complex cases

W. Stuart Reynolds & Roger R. Dmochowski

Key points

- In patients with mixed urinary incontinence, prioritising the most bothersome component (stress or urgency urinary incontinence) will help to direct initial primary therapy.
- Urinary sphincter damage during prostatectomy is the primary cause of incontinence in men after prostatectomy and can be treated effectively with an artificial urinary sphincter or male sling procedure.
- Concomitant urinary incontinence and pelvic organ prolapse is common in women; occult or undiagnosed stress urinary incontinence can often be demonstrated in women with significant prolapse and no subjective complaints of incontinence, either on pre-operative prolapse reduction testing or after prolapse treatment.
- Treatment for neurogenic overactive bladder syndrome should be directed by findings on pretreatment testing (e.g. urodynamics) and often requires modification and re-assessment over time as the neurologic process evolves and long-term bladder changes develop.
- A multidisciplinary perspective on urinary incontinence in elderly patients can help identify many potential contributory factors that are not directly related to the genitourinary system, but may have significant impacts on continence care.

6.1 **Introduction**

Complex cases of urinary incontinence can prove to be difficult situations for healthcare providers, as a number of aspects related to an individual patient's overall circumstance influence the nature and degree of incontinence. Determining the specific nature of incontinence, whether related to activity or abdominal straining i.e. stress urinary incontinence (SUI) or related to urgency i.e. urgency urinary incontinence (UUI) as part of the overactive bladder (OAB), may be problematic because of difficulty distinguishing different symptoms, as in the case of mixed urinary incontinence (MUI). Patient factors, such as comorbid medical conditions, neurological disorders, and previous pelvic and urinary tract surgeries may also complicate the diagnosis and treatment of incontinence.

In many of these difficult situations, advanced testing of lower urinary tract function is warranted to better delineate signs and symptoms and to direct treatment approaches.

Multichannel urodynamics is the preferred method for testing lower urinary tract function and should be considered in any case that may be complex, especially prior to initiating surgical treatment.

6.2 **Mixed urinary incontinence**

Urinary incontinence often represents a spectrum of lower urinary tract dysfunction related to physiological and anatomical abnormalities of the genitourinary system. When UUI, associated with urgency and frequency, as part of OAB, coexists with incontinence associated with activity or valsalva (SUI), then the condition is referred to as mixed urinary incontinence (MUI). The relative contribution of each component of incontinence (i.e. SUI and UUI) can vary in individual patients and the symptoms often overlap, making distinctions between the two difficult.

In the majority of cases of urinary incontinence, mixed urinary incontinence is present to varying degrees, and the relative contribution of each component (SUI and UUI) needs to be assessed.

6.2.2 **Treatment considerations for mixed urinary incontinence**

Treatment of MUI poses many dilemmas for the healthcare provider, as both components of MUI (i.e. SUI and UUI) are treated differently from each other. In order to best approach this dilemma, the doctor or nurse must help the patient prioritize the bothersome symptoms and consider treating the most bothersome first.

Further testing modalities, particular multichannel urodynamics, may be needed to better delineate the contributory aspects of SUI and UUI to MUI and guide therapeutic strategies.

6.2.3 Stress urinary incontinence surgery in the setting of mixed urinary incontinence

Surgical treatment of SUI in the setting of MUI is an appropriate initial approach, but several aspects need to be considered. In a patient with SUI-predominant MUI, outcomes are varied after surgical intervention:

- In general, a decreased overall efficacy of SUI surgery can be expected when MUI exists as compared with pure SUI, although stress incontinence-specific improvements may be uniform
- In many situations, OAB symptoms including UUI can be improved or cured with surgery for SUI in up to 75% of patients.

A subsequent improvement in OAB symptoms after SUI surgery may be related to reversing the phenomenon of reflex excitation of the bladder due an incompetent bladder neck that allows urine into the proximal urethra. By improving coaptation of the bladder neck and proximal urethra, urine may not lie in the proximal urethra after surgical intervention, and the reflex excitation of the bladder is eliminated and the OAB symptoms cured or improved.

New additional symptoms of frequency and urgency (termed 'de novo urgency') can also develop after surgery for SUI in up to 30% of patients, although many patients may have had OAB symptoms that were unrecorded or underplayed before surgery. Some believe that de novo urgency may develop from iatrogenic, relative urethral obstruction after surgical SUI treatment, although the exact aetiology remains unknown. Patients undergoing SUI surgery need to be counselled both about the possible persistence of OAB symptoms and their potential development, as de novo OAB.

Urinary symptoms related to OAB including UUI can be treated either before, or after SUI surgery if they persist, with the usual interventions for OAB, including anticholinergic medications.

6.2.4 Pharmacological treatment of mixed urinary incontinence

Anticholinergic medications are the primary mode for treating OAB symptoms including UUI, even in the setting of MUI. In patients with UUI predominant MUI, a trial of anticholinergic medications is warranted. Additional treatment options for OAB symptoms may also be employed as needed, if anticholinergic therapy fails, such as botulinum toxin injection or sacral nerve stimulation.

Antidepressants

Tricyclic antidepressants (TCA) are potentially useful agents for treating MUI because of their multitude of actions on the nervous system: direct anticholinergic effects, inhibition of norepinephrine and serotonin reuptake at nerve terminals, and sedative effects. In the setting of MUI, TCAs can both decrease bladder contractility and increase outlet resistance, providing symptomatic relief for both components of MUI.

The most well known TCA for urinary conditions is imipramine, which has been shown clinically to effectively decrease bladder contractility and increase bladder outlet resistance.

At daily doses of 25–75 mg, benefits and cures can be seen up to 30–70% of patients with incontinence. Used in conjunction with an anticholinergic medication, the effects on bladder contractility are additive; however, the side effect profiles are also additive. Rarely, serious side effects can occur related to cardiac toxicity and central nervous system effects, so using imipramine should be done so with caution.

Duloxetine, a serotonin and norepinephrine reuptake inhibitor has also been used for the treatment of MUI. It has actions similar to TCA in that it increases sphincteric muscle activity and decreases bladder contractility. Clinical evidence reveals marginal improvements over placebo, particularly in SUI symptoms; however, the medication is not currently available in the United States.

6.3 Post-prostatectomy incontinence

6.3.1 Epidemiology of post-prostatectomy incontinence

Urinary incontinence after prostatectomy is a known complication of the procedure and occurs anywhere from 0 to 65% of men undergoing prostatectomy. The severity of post-prostatectomy incontinence (PPI) can range from a small amount of leakage with abdominal straining, valsalva or activity in most men to florid, total incontinence in a minority of men. Characterizing and quantifying the degree of urinary leakage after prostatectomy has been historically difficult and controversial, depending on the definition of incontinence and method used to ascertain the outcome (e.g. patient self-reported vs. physician assessment). Additionally, objectifying the degree of psychological bother caused by PPI has also been inconsistent and problematic:

- On average, approximately 20% of men will report moderate or daily incontinence, with 5–10% reporting significant or total incontinence
- Recovery of continence after prostatectomy is generally progressive: most men will be incontinent immediately after surgery

and urinary control will improve for up to 24 months, with the greatest improvement in the initial three to nine months
- Between 2 and 6% of men after prostatectomy will undergo subsequent surgical treatment for PPI.

6.3.2 Pathophysiology of post-prostatectomy incontinence

In men with PPI, an abnormality of the urinary sphincter is the main cause of incontinence. In the normal male, the urinary sphincter mechanism is comprised of two functionally distinct units: the proximal and distal urethral sphincters. The proximal sphincter consists of the bladder neck, prostate and prostatic urethra. The distal urethral sphincter is a complex of structures including the rhabdosphincter (external sphincter muscle), the extrinsic para-urethral musculature, and the intrinsic urethral tissue. During prostatectomy, the proximal urethral sphincter is removed with the prostate specimen, leaving only the distal urethral sphincter mechanism to maintain continence. The degree to which this sole remaining mechanism can maintain continence is variable and largely dependent on the individual. Damage to and/or fibrosis of the distal sphincter support mechanism may additionally contribute poor sphincter function.

In some cases, bladder dysfunction in addition to sphincter insufficiency may contribute to PPI. Bladder overactivity and decreased bladder compliance occur in conjunction with sphincter deficiency in up to a third of patients with PPI, although rarely without concomitant sphincter insufficiency. Multichannel urodynamics are therefore recommended for the evaluation of PPI before surgical intervention.

6.3.3 Treatment options for post-prostatectomy incontinence

Pelvic floor muscle training (i.e. Kegel exercises) may improve continence marginally and any benefit is seen primarily in the early postoperative period (<3 months). There are no pharmacological options for PPI, unless bladder dysfunction (i.e. overactive bladder) is present in conjunction with sphincter dysfunction. For men with persistent PPI, the primary mode of treatment is surgical.

The primary surgical treatment modalities for PPI include the male urethral sling and the artificial urinary sphincter (AUS).

Male sling

For the male sling procedure, a graft material, either biological or synthetic (e.g. polypropylene mesh), is surgically implanted under the proximal bulbar urethra to apply compressive force to the urethra as well as to support the urethral sphincter mechanism. This compressive force functionally obstructs the urethra, resulting in urinary continence during rest, as well as during abdominal straining. Several methods have been established to secure the mesh, including bone anchors affixed to the under-surface of the pubic bone as well as suspending the graft material by looping it around bony structures (i.e. transobturator slings):

- Continence can be achieved in the majority of patients (50–80%) after male sling procedure, particularly in men with mild and moderate degrees of incontinence, although 'mild' and 'moderate' are not defined, as yet
- For men with significant or severe PPI, a male sling may not be as successful in achieving continence as in milder degrees of leakage.

Artificial urinary sphincter

Urinary incontinence after prostatectomy is most effectively treated with an AUS, which is a surgically implanted medical device designed to obstruct the proximal urethra in the closed state during urine storage and to allow urine passage in the open state during voiding.

The present configuration of the AUS is comprised of three functional, contiguous components: the circumferential urethral cuff, the pump mechanism, and the pressure-regulating balloon (PRB) or reservoir.

The urethral cuff is implanted at the level of the proximal bulbar urethra and wraps completely around the urethra. The pump is implanted in the dependent scrotum and the PRB in the abdominal cavity. The entire device is filled with sterile saline at the time of implantation; the inherent mechanics of the device maintain a constant fluid pressure across the components of the device. Pressure is delivered to the urethral cuff through the transmission of a fluid column generated passively from the PRB. Manipulating the pump effectively opens and closes the urethral cuff:

- In the resting or closed state, the cuff applies a constant, circumferential pressure to the urethra to effectively stop urine leakage
- When voiding is desired, the pump is manually activated ('pumped'), driving the fluid out of the cuff and back to the PRB, relieving the occluding pressure from the urethra and allowing the urine to flow normally
- The fluid then cycles passively back into the cuff over 60–90 seconds from the PRB and the urethral pressure or continence mechanism is reestablished.

Success (as measured by the degree of dryness) after AUS implantation is generally reported up to 90%, and patient satisfaction also rates consistently up to 90%, even when total continence is not achieved. These favourable results are hampered somewhat by the negative impact of device complications requiring revision, replacement or removal, including device malfunction/failure, urethral atrophy, infection and erosion. The overall 5-year expected device survival (i.e. no revisions) is estimated at 75%, while long-term efficacy has been demonstrated over 10–15 years.

6.4 Pelvic organ prolapse

6.4.1 Association of urinary incontinence and pelvic organ prolapse

Urinary incontinence, particularly SUI, is a common associated finding with pelvic organ prolapse (POP) and reflects a commonality of pelvic floor disorders related to the failure of anatomic structures supporting the pelvic organs. Just as loss of the support mechanisms and structures for the vagina result in POP, loss of the support mechanisms for the bladder neck and urethra result in SUI.

- SUI occurs in up to 40% of patients with symptomatic POP
- Urinary urgency as part of overactive bladder has been reported in up to 33% of women with symptomatic POP
- SUI generally requires specific surgical correction for resolution and surgical repair of POP, but this does not necessarily treat concurrent SUI
- Surgical correction of POP often can improve or cure urinary urgency
- In women without previous SUI undergoing POP repair, up to 60% may develop new or de novo SUI after POP treatment.

6.4.2 Occult stress urinary incontinence

The degree of urinary incontinence can be related to the severity of POP. As the degree of POP worsens, the amount of SUI can paradoxically diminish as the prolapsing organs and bladder effectively 'kink off' the urethra and produce a functional obstruction of the urethra at the level of the bladder neck. Patients may not complain of urinary incontinence at all or, more commonly, may report that previous urinary incontinence has improved as the POP has worsened. Ultimately, enough urethral obstruction may develop such that the woman may not be able to voluntarily void at all or empty her bladder efficiently. When the POP is reduced, either temporarily with physical examination or vaginal splint (e.g. pessary) or permanently with surgical correction, the SUI may be un-masked and easily demonstrated once the kinking is removed:

- SUI that is only demonstrable by reducing POP is referred to as 'occult stress incontinence'
- Occult SUI can be demonstrated in 30–80% of women with POP

• Detecting occult SUI may be important for counselling patients prior to surgical correction of POP as well as for planning for concurrent treatment of SUI at the time of POP repair.

6.4.3 **Treatment strategies**

Treatment of urinary incontinence associated with POP may proceed through a variety of surgical techniques and approaches, which have been described elsewhere. Several different strategies may be employed when considering surgical treatment of concurrent SUI and POP. In patients with demonstrable SUI and POP, surgical treatment of POP, at the same time as SUI repair (particularly with a mid-urethral sling), does not adversely affect the cure rate for SUI. This may be the preferred treatment strategy for women presenting with known SUI and those with occult SUI demonstrable on pre-operative reduction testing. For continent women with POP, including those in whom occult SUI was not demonstrated on pre-operative testing, either prophylactic anti-incontinence procedures can be performed at the time of POP repair or POP can proceed without anti-incontinence procedures and de novo SUI can be subsequently treated at a later time with an additional procedure:

• Prophylactic anti-incontinence procedures performed at the time of POP surgery can prevent the need for subsequent anti-incontinence surgery in women who may develop de novo SUI, but may subject more women to the complications and morbidity associated with the procedures

• Avoiding prophylactic anti-incontinence surgery at the time of POP repair will necessitate subjecting those women who develop bothersome de novo SUI to another surgical procedure; however, it will avoid subjecting women who do not develop SUI to the adverse consequences of the procedure.

6.5 **Neurogenic overactive bladder syndrome**

6.5.1 **Evaluation and assessment**

Individual patient characteristics and clinical situations, as well as urinary tract symptoms, must all be assessed when evaluating a patient with either a known or suspected neurogenic voiding abnormality, including OAB. Neurological aetiologies for lower urinary tract (LUT) dysfunction manifest in many different functional aspects, which may collectively present with common urinary complaints. Additionally, unfavourable LUT function can result in major detrimental medical situations (e.g. renal dysfunction and failure, and pyelonephritis and sepsis) that can be prevented with proper assessment and treatment. Therefore, defining the underlying LUT dysfunction is important for directing management approaches.

Assessment of lower urinary tract function

Multichannel urodynamics should be a cornerstone of evaluation for patients with neurogenic OAB, as significant bladder abnormalities can be uncovered, which often dictate various treatment options. Several specific components of the testing procedure are necessary for assessment, including cystometrogram (CMG) and pressure-flow studies (PFS), with electromyography (EMG) and fluoroscopic imaging being additional, informative components. Common findings on urodynamics that may influence the treatment approach include the presence of detrusor overactivity (DO) with or without associated DO incontinence, stress incontinence with provocative manoeuvres, changes in bladder compliance, decreased bladder capacity, elevated resting bladder pressures, poor contractility, and ineffective voiding or emptying (e.g. obstruction, detrusor-sphincter dysynergia, elevated post-void residual).

- A comprehensive assessment of LUT function should be performed at initial patient presentation and prior to initiating empiric therapy
- Changes or progression in neurological status or clinical changes in voiding function should prompt reassessment of LUT function.

Additional testing

Additional testing may be warranted in some cases of neurogenic OAB, including imaging to evaluate structural aspects of the kidneys and spine. Renal sonography or ultrasound is an excellent, non-invasive radiographic study to evaluate the structure and configuration of upper urinary tract components, including the kidneys and ureters. Ureteral dilation, hydronephrosis of the kidney, and qualitative assessment of the renal cortex are all factors that can provide clues to the presence or risk of progressive renal dysfunction. Spinal magnetic resonance imaging (MRI) may be considered in some patients who present with findings of neurogenic LUT dysfunction in order to determine a neurological aetiological factor, if no previous diagnosis has been made.

6.5.2 Treatment considerations

Considerations of patient expectations and goals should be integrated with overlying aspects of neurological disease prognosis. Depending on the neurological aetiology and condition, selecting appropriate treatment strategies must consider long-term goals and expectations as well. Evolution of degenerative neurological processes, progressive, irreversible LUT dysfunction, and changing environments and caregiver availability are but a few examples of dynamic aspects of care that mandate re-evaluation of current and proposed treatment options.

6.5.3 Treatment options for neurogenic overactive bladder syndrome

As discussed above, treatment options for neurogenic OAB will depend on the underlying nature of the neurological condition and the over-riding functional ability and expectations of the individual patient. Pharmacological, neuromodulation, and invasive surgery are all viable treatment options for appropriate patients.

Pharmacological therapy

The mainstay class of medications for pharmacological treatment of neurogenic OAB are the anticholinergic agents, which diminish the frequency and amplitude of involuntary detrusor contractions, characteristic of DO, and which increase bladder compliance and capacity. Anticholinergics can often be used in conjunction with other treatment modalities, including, for instance, intermittent self-catheterization (ISC), which is used for inefficient bladder emptying.

Neuromodulation therapy

Neuromodulation therapy is typically reserved for patients failing primary therapy with oral agents (e.g. anticholinergics) and behaviour modifications, if appropriate. Neuromodulation collectively includes toxin-mediated modulation of the bladder as well as peripheral nerve stimulation.

Botulinum toxin therapy

Botulinum toxin (BoTN) therapy for the bladder in patients with neurogenic OAB is a minimally invasive, but highly effective treatment option for refractory OAB and voiding complaints. BoTN is produced by the bacterium *clostridium botulinum*, the causative agent in the disease botulism, and while lethal in toxic doses, can be therapeutic at significantly lower concentrations. BoTN blocks the release of acetylcholine from motor nerve fibres at the neuromuscular junction (the junction between nerve and muscle fibres), effectively causing muscle paralysis. Bladder muscle paralysis results in decreased frequency and amplitude of involuntary detrusor contractions while also increasing bladder capacity and compliance, resulting in decreased resting bladder pressures. While several subtypes of BoTN exist, it is primarily sub-type A that is used clinically in medical therapy (BTA).

BTA is easily injected into the wall of the bladder from within the lumen using standard urological endoscopic equipment (i.e. cystoscopy) and can be accomplished in an outpatient setting with minimal sedation or in the office after instillation of local anaesthetic into the bladder. A range of dosing options is available, with typical doses ranging from 50 to 300 units in total; spread over 15–30 separate bladder injections. The higher the dose, the more effective the treatment; however, the greatest side effect of BTA injection is urinary retention, which must be weighed against the clinical benefits. Many patients with neurogenic LUT dysfunction are already catheter-dependent because of incomplete bladder emptying (i.e. on ISC), so the highest effective dose (300 units) is typically administered in this situation, as the consequences of urinary retention is negligible. Unfortunately, the clinical benefits of BTA injection are time dependent and tend to wear off after approximately 6 months, at which time re-injection is necessary.

Peripheral nerve stimulation

Neuromodulation by manipulating or stimulating peripheral nerves can also be used for the treatment of DO in neurogenic bladder patients. Sacral nerve modulation or stimulation (SNS) is the most popular and common procedure related to bladder abnormalities, but pudendal nerve stimulation, genital nerve stimulation and posterior tibial nerve stimulation have all been used for treatment of bladder dysfunction. The exact mechanism that leads to SNS being effective has yet to be elucidated; however, therapeutic effects on bladder function are seen when the sacral nerve roots, particularly at S3 spinal level, are electrically stimulated with low amplitude shocks. A SNS device is comprised of two components: an electric stimulator lead and an electrical impulse generator (IPG). The entire device is surgically implanted under the skin, with the electric stimulator lead inserted into the S3 spinal foramen adjacent to the S3 nerve root and the IPG implanted in upper buttock region. The IPG can be remotely programmed and the amplitude of the electrical impulses manipulated to maximize effect.

- Sacral nerve stimulation can be used in the settings of OAB/DO with or without incontinence as well as for some cases of urinary retention
- In the setting of neurogenic bladder, a limiting aspect of SNS are the spinal deformities and irregularities that may be prohibitive of proper, safe placement
- An implanted SNS device is a contraindication for MRI, which may be a limitation to neurological disease diagnosis and evaluation. If it is anticipated that a patient will need MRIs, then SNS is not a viable option for that patient.

Surgical intervention

When less invasive management options for neurogenic OAB have failed, more drastic surgical options may be necessary. Involuntary detrusor contractions (DO) with urine leakage, small bladder capacity, low compliance, and elevated bladder resting pressures can all be effectively treated by physically increasing the size of the bladder through an augmentation procedure. A bladder augmentation involves surgically placing a 'patch' constructed from bowel (typically small intestine) on the bladder, thereby increasing the capacity (and compliance) while at the same time disrupting some of the mechanisms that generate detrusor contractions. This is a major operation, requiring hospitalization and significant recovery. In addition, effective emptying of the bladder will be eliminated and a patient undergoing bladder augmentation will by necessity be dependent on ISC to empty the bladder. Nevertheless, the results can be excellent after augmentation, with significantly improved continence and overall urinary tract function.

In some patients, where dependence on ISC can be problematic due to functional limitations and caregiver issues, total urinary diversion is an acceptable and reasonable option. In addition, in advanced cases of pressure wound breakdown and urine soiling, urinary diversion may be the best strategy. The most popular version of urinary diversion is an ideal conduit or urostomy, which involves surgically re-routing the urine passage from the kidneys and ureters to the abdominal wall skin, via a 'conduit' of small intestine (i.e. ileum), to be collected in an external appliance or bag. Although this too is a major surgical procedure, the results can be excellent and literally, life changing.

6.6 Elderly patients

6.6.1 Multi-factorial aspects of urinary incontinence in elderly

Urinary incontinence in the elderly is a complex entity, usually with roots well beyond the LUT. Often the aetiology of incontinence is multi-factorial or multi-dimensional involving multiple interacting risk factors, including age-related physiological changes and comorbidity, as well as LUT pathology. Additionally, the impact and resulting functional impairment of urinary incontinence on the elderly has broader implications than for younger adults, and extends to caregivers and the greater society at large. Treatment considerations must take into account these broader aspects of the condition in the older patient.

Urinary incontinence in the elderly may be considered a geriatric syndrome, as many risk factors are not directly related to the genitourinary tract, but contribute to the overall burden of disease.

Age-related changes to genitourinary tract
Age-related physiological changes can contribute to, but rarely cause urinary incontinence alone. Often pathological changes in

the urinary tract are magnified by the contribution of physiological changes. Age-related changes to the genitourinary tract that may have implications for urinary incontinence are listed in Table 6.1.

Table 6.1 Age-related physiological changes related to urinary incontinence
Bladder function   • Decreased capacity   • Increased overactivity   • Decreased contractility   • Increased residual urine
Urethra   Decreased intrinsic function
Prostate   • Developing benign prostatic obstruction   • Increased prostate cancer
Hormonal factors   Decreased oestrogen
Increased night-time urine production
Altered central and peripheral neurological factors
Altered immune function

Comorbid conditions and factors associated with risks of urinary incontinence

Factors beyond the urinary system significantly contribute to the syndrome of urinary incontinence in the elderly. Comorbid medical illnesses, neurological, and psychiatric disorders, medications, functional impairments and environmental factors are all potential risk factors for the development and potentiation of urinary incontinence within the concept of the syndrome. Specific comorbid conditions and factors are listed in Table 6.2.

6.6.2 **Causes of transient incontinence**

Transient causes of urinary incontinence are very common in the elderly population, accounting for one-third cases of incontinence in the community-dwelling elderly, up to one-half of cases of acute hospitalizations and greater proportion of nursing home admissions. Consistent with the concept of geriatric syndrome, transient causes of urinary incontinence are most often not directly related to the genitourinary system:

Table 6.2 Conditions and factors contributing to urinary incontinence in elderly

Comorbid medical illnesses
- Diabetes mellitus
- Degenerative joint disease
- Chronic pulmonary disease
- Congestive heart failure
- Lower extremity oedema
- Sleep apnoea
- Constipation and stool impaction

Neurological and psychiatric disorders
- Stroke
- Parkinson's disease
- Dementia/Alzheimer's disease
- Depression

Medications
- Alpha-adrenergic agonists and antagonists
- Angiotensin-converting enzyme inhibitors
- Anticholinergics
- Calcium-channel blockers
- Cholinesterase inhibitors
- Diuretics
- Lithium
- Opioid analgesics
- Psychotropic agents (including sedatives and anxiolytics, hypnotics, antipsychotics)
- Selective serotonin re-uptake inhibitors
- Others (gabapentin, glitazones, non-steroidal anti-inflammatory drugs)

Functional impairments
- Impaired mobility
- Impaired cognition

Environment factors
- Inaccessible toilets
- Unavailable caregivers

- Transient causes of incontinence in the elderly can be categorized according to the mnemonic DIAPPERS (see Table 6.3)
- Modification or resolution of causes of transient incontinence will generally restore continence or improve it.

Table 6.3	**Causes of transient urinary incontinence in elderly patients**
D	Delirium
I	Infection
A	Atrophic urethritis/vaginitis
P	Psychological (e.g. depression, neurosis)
P	Pharmacological
E	Excess urine production
R	Restricted mobility
S	Stool impaction

6.6.3 Treatment considerations

Treating urinary incontinence in the elderly population must address the various components of the overall syndrome and often entails contributions from several healthcare providers involved in an individual's care. Often modifying or improving some of the ancillary factors not directly involving the genitourinary system can improve the associated incontinence. Management of specific comorbid conditions, improvement and modification of environmental factors, and addressing functional impairments are all aspects with potential utility for incontinence treatment, and which involve various aspects of a multidisciplinary, team-based approach.

A multidisciplinary approach or perspective on an individual basis can help to identify any number of potential factors contributing to urinary incontinence that can be managed effectively and simply with significant impact on continence.

Other general considerations regarding treatment of incontinence in elderly relate to defining appropriate outcomes and goals of therapy, while considering life expectancy, preferences for care, and the costs and benefits of specific treatment modalities. Additionally, pharmacological issues need to be considered relative to polypharmacy concerns and drug interactions, age-related changes in pharmacokinetics and drug metabolism, and the frequency and impact of adverse drug effects.

6.6.4 Treatment modalities

Several modalities are available for the treatment of urinary incontinence in the elderly, including lifestyle and behavioural interventions, pharmacological therapy, and surgical intervention.

Lifestyle and behavioural modifications

Modifying lifestyle and behavioural habits has the benefit of inducing few adverse effects, while potentially significantly impacting not only on urinary incontinence, but also on other aspects of an individual's health condition as well. Fluid management (both preventing dehydration, as well as fluid excess) can mitigate some the aspects of incontinence, while avoiding dietary stimulants (e.g. caffeine) can reduce OAB symptoms. Encouraging a well-balanced diet can improve constipation and bowel habits, whilst contributing to weight loss, increased energy and thus activity, potentially improving functional impairments which may be an impediment to maintaining continence.

Voiding-specific behaviour modifications can also improve voiding and continence, and include prompted voiding, habit training, timed voiding, and combined toileting and exercise therapy. Caregiver participation, if relevant, is important to implementing behaviour therapies.

Pharmacological therapy

Pharmacological intervention for urinary incontinence and OAB in elderly patients generally mirrors that in younger aged groups, with the caveat that increased consideration be given to addressing and preventing potential adverse effects and drug-drug interactions. Anticholinergic medications are still the preferred pharmacological class of medications for OAB because of their efficacy in controlling symptoms.

Concerns over cognitive and sedative effects of anticholinergic medications, particularly in the elderly, have been validated, and selecting appropriate agents for OAB therapy must address this issue.

Some anticholinergics, because of the selectivity profile or molecular profile, have been demonstrated to have less cognitive effects on patients than others (e.g. darifenacin, trospium), and these should be considered first in initiating therapy. Age-related physiological changes in drug metabolism and issues of polypharmacy, as well as adverse effects, all reinforce the fact that a conservative approach should be used when initiating anticholinergic therapy with assessment and awareness of these factors.

Starting with a lower dose and slowly titrating to effect, while being mindful of adverse effects, is the recommended approach and mirrors the common axiom, 'start low and go slow.'

Surgical intervention

Surgical treatment options for urinary incontinence in the elderly remain similar to those available in younger age groups. Most controlled studies involving surgical treatments for incontinence have traditionally not included elderly patients as trial participants, so high quality clinical evidence for efficacy of treatments in elderly patients is lacking. Nevertheless, most treatment options remain possible to elderly patients with incontinence.

Surgical morbidity in the elderly is generally related to overall health issues, comorbid medical conditions and functional impairments rather than to specific aspects of incontinence procedures.

The risks of morbidity and mortality, otherwise, are similar for elderly patients as for younger patients.

Considerations regarding goals and expectations of treatment outcomes as well as longevity need to be addressed prior to surgical intervention, in addition to the incontinence and voiding situations. Trading long-term efficacy for decreased morbidity and recovery may be an appropriate approach in elderly patients, and treatments such as urethral bulking agents for SUI may be preferred in this setting. Relatively less-invasive SUI procedures such as mid-urethral synthetic slings may also be considered, as both the morbidity and recovery appear favourable in most populations.

Key references

Abrams P, Andersson KE, Birder L, Brubaker L, Cardozo L, Chapple C, *et al.* (2010). Fourth international consultation on incontinence recommendations of the international scientific committee: Evaluation and treatment of urinary incontinence, pelvic organ prolapse, and faecal incontinence. *Neurourol. Urodyn,* **29**, 213–40.

Brubaker L, Glazener C, Jacquentin B, Maher C, Melgrem A, Norton P, *et al.* (2009). Surgery for Pelvic Organ Prolapse in Abrams P, Cardozo L, Khoury S and Wein A, eds., *Incontinence: 4th International Consultation on Incontinence,* 4th edn. Paris: Health Publication Ltd, 1273–320.

Casanova N, McGuire E, Fenner DE (2006). Botulinum toxin: a potential alternative to current treatment of neurogenic and idiopathic urinary incontinence due to detrusor overactivity. *Int J Gynaecol Obstet,* **95**, 305–11.

Comiter CV (2007). Surgery insight: surgical management of postprostatectomy incontinence: the artificial urinary sphincter and male sling. *Nat Clin Pract Urol,* **4**, 615–24.

Dmochowski RR, Blaivas JM, Gormley EA, Juma S, Karram MM, Lightner DJ, *et al.* (2010). Update of AUA guideline on the surgical management of female stress urinary incontinence. *J Urol,* **183**, 1906–11.

DuBeau CE, Kuchel GA, Johnson T, Palmer MH, Wagg A (2009). Incontinence in the frail elderly. In: Abrams P, Cardozo L, Khoury S, Wein AJ, (eds) *Incontinence: 4th International Consultation on Incontinence.* Paris: Health Publication Ltd, 691–1024.

McGuire E J (2010). Urodynamics of the neurogenic bladder. *Urol Clin North Am,* **37**, 507–16.

Peters KM (2010). Alternative approaches to sacral nerve stimulation. *Int Urogynecol J Pelvic Floor Dysfunct,* **21**, 1559–63.

Singh G, Lucas M, Dolan L, Knight S, Ramage C, Hobson PT (2010). Minimum standards for urodynamic practice in the UK. *Neurourol Urodyn,* **29**, 1365–72.

Smith T, Chang D, Dmochowski R, Hilton P, Nilsson CG, Reid FM, *et al.* (2009). Surgery for urinary incontinence in women. In: Abrams P, Cardozo L, Khoury S, Wein AJ (eds), *Incontinence: 4th International Consultation on Incontinence.* Paris: Health Publications Ltd, 1191–272.

Appendix

International Consultation and National Institute for Health and Clinical Excellence (NICE) guidelines

Hashim Hashim & Paul Abrams

1 NICE storage lower urinary tract symptoms guidelines for men

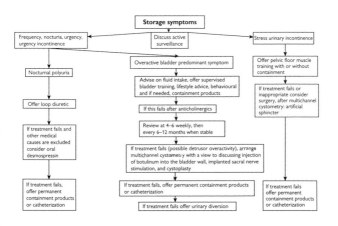

```
                              Storage symptoms

Frequency, nocturia, urgency,        Discuss active              Stress urinary incontinence
urgency incontinence                 surveillance

                                                                 Offer pelvic floor muscle
                                                                 training with or without
    Nocturnal polyuria      Overactive bladder predominant symptom    containment

                            Advise on fluid intake, offer supervised   If treatment fails or
    Offer loop diuretic     bladder training, lifestyle advice, behavioural   inappropriate consider
                            and if needed, containment products      surgery, after multichannel
                                                                 cystometry: artificial
    If treatment fails and  If this fails after anticholinergics    sphincter
    other medical
    causes are excluded     Review at 4–6 weekly, then
    consider oral           every 6–12 months when stable
    desmopressin
                            If treatment fails (possible detrusor overactivity), arrange
                            multichannel cystometry with a view to discussing injection
                            of botulinum into the bladder wall, implanted sacral nerve
                            stimulation, and cystoplasty

    If treatment fails,     If treatment fails, offer permanent containment products   If treatment fails
    offer permanent         or catheterization                        offer permanent
    containment products                                             containment products
    or catheterization      If treatment fails offer urinary diversion   or catheterization
```

Reproduced from: National Clinical Guideline Centre (2010). *Lower urinary tract symptoms: the management of lower urinary tract symptoms in men.* London: National Clinical Guideline Centre.

2 International Consultation on Prostate Disease guidelines for lower urinary tract symptoms in men

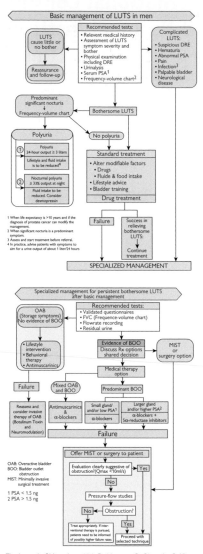

Reprinted from *The Journal of Neurology*, **181**, P. Abrams, C. Chapple, S. Khoury, C. Roehrborn, J. de la Rosette. Evaluation and treatment of lower urinary tract symptoms in older men, 1779–1787, (2009), with permission from Elsevier.

3 International Consultation on Incontinence guidelines for men

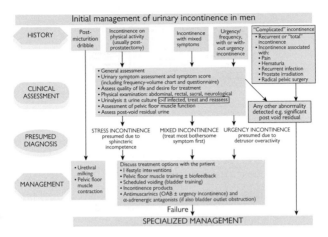

Initial management of urinary incontinence in men

HISTORY — Post-micturition dribble | Incontinence on physical activity (usually post-prostatectomy) | Incontinence with mixed symptoms | Urgency/frequency, with or without urgency incontinence | "Complicated" incontinence
• Recurrent or "total" incontinence
• Incontinence associated with:
  • Pain
  • Hematuria
  • Recurrent infection
  • Prostate irradiation
  • Radical pelvic surgery

CLINICAL ASSESSMENT
• General assessment
• Urinary symptom assessment and symptom score (including frequency-volume chart and questionnaire)
• Assess quality of life and desire for treatment
• Physical examination: abdominal, rectal, sacral, neurological
• Urinalysis ± urine culture >if infected, treat and reassess
• Assessment of pelvic floor muscle function
• Assess post-void residual urine

Any other abnormality detected e.g. significant post void residual

PRESUMED DIAGNOSIS — STRESS INCONTINENCE presumed due to sphincteric incompetence | MIXED INCONTINENCE (treat most bothersome symptom first) | URGENCY INCONTINENCE presumed due to detrusor overactivity

MANAGEMENT
• Urethral milking
• Pelvic floor muscle contraction

Discuss treatment options with the patient
• Lifestyle interventions
• Pelvic floor muscle training ± biofeedback
• Scheduled voiding (bladder training)
• Incontinence products
• Antimuscarinics (OAB ± urgency incontinence) and α-adrenergic antagonists (if also bladder outlet obstruction)

Failure ↓

SPECIALIZED MANAGEMENT

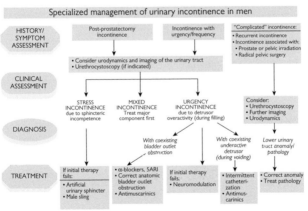

Specialized management of urinary incontinence in men

HISTORY/ SYMPTOM ASSESSMENT — Post-prostatectomy incontinence | Incontinence with urgency/frequency | "Complicated" incontinence:
• Recurrent incontinence
• Incontinence associated with:
  • Prostate or pelvic irradiation
  • Radical pelvic surgery

CLINICAL ASSESSMENT
• Consider urodynamics and imaging of the urinary tract
• Urethrocystoscopy (if indicated)

DIAGNOSIS — STRESS INCONTINENCE due to sphincteric incompetence | MIXED INCONTINENCE Treat major component first | URGENCY INCONTINENCE due to detrusor overactivity (during filling) | Consider:
• Urethrocystoscopy
• Further imaging
• Urodynamics

With coexisting bladder outlet obstruction | With coexisting underactive detrusor (during voiding) | Lower urinary tract anomaly/ pathology

TREATMENT
If initial therapy fails:
• Artificial urinary sphincter
• Male sling

• α-blockers, 5ARI
• Correct anatomic bladder outlet obstruction
• Antimuscarinics

If initial therapy fails:
• Neuromodulation

• Intermittent catheterization
• Antimuscarinics

• Correct anomaly
• Treat pathology

4 NICE Overactive Bladder/Urgency Urinary Incontinence guidelines for women

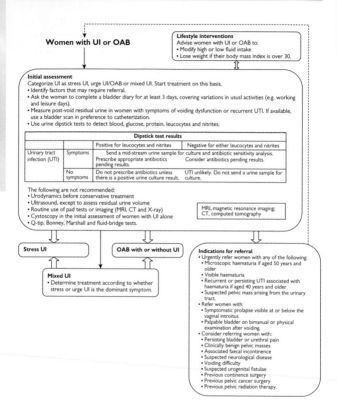

Women with UI or OAB

Lifestyle interventions
Advise women with UI or OAB to:
• Modify high or low fluid intake
• Lose weight if their body mass index is over 30.

Initial assessment
Categorize UI as stress UI, urge UI/OAB or mixed UI. Start treatment on this basis.
• Identify factors that may require referral.
• Ask the woman to complete a bladder diary for at least 3 days, covering variations in usual activities (e.g. working and leisure days).
• Measure post-void residual urine in women with symptoms of voiding dysfunction or recurrent UTI. If available, use a bladder scan in preference to catheterization.
• Use urine dipstick tests to detect blood, glucose, protein, leucocytes and nitrites.

		Dipstick test results	
		Positive for leucocytes and nitrites	Negative for either leucocytes and nitrites
Urinary tract infection (UTI)	Symptoms	Send a mid-stream urine sample for culture and antibiotic sensitivity analysis. Prescribe appropriate antibiotics pending results.	Consider antibiotics pending results.
	No symptoms	Do not prescribe antibiotics unless there is a positive urine culture result.	UTI unlikely. Do not send a urine sample for culture.

The following are not recommended:
• Urodynamics before conservative treatment
• Ultrasound, except to assess residual urine volume
• Routine use of pad tests or imaging (MRI, CT and X-ray)
• Cystoscopy in the initial assessment of women with UI alone
• Q-tip, Bonney, Marshall and fluid-bridge tests.

MRI, magnetic resonance imaging; CT, computed tomography

Stress UI

OAB with or without UI

Mixed UI
• Determine treatment according to whether stress or urge UI is the dominant symptom.

Indications for referral
• Urgently refer women with any of the following:
  • Microscopic haematuria if aged 50 years and older
  • Visible haematuria
  • Recurrent or persisting UTI associated with haematuria if aged 40 years and older
  • Suspected pelvic mass arising from the urinary tract.
• Refer women with:
  • Symptomatic prolapse visible at or below the vaginal introitus
  • Palpable bladder on bimanual or physical examination after voiding.
• Consider referring women with:
  • Persisting bladder or urethral pain
  • Clinically benign pelvic masses
  • Associated faecal incontinence
  • Suspected neurological disease
  • Voiding difficulty
  • Suspected urogenital fistulae
  • Previous continence surgery
  • Previous pelvic cancer surgery
  • Previous pelvic radiation therapy.

Reproduced with permission of the Royal College of Obstetricians and Gynaecologists.

5 NICE Stress Urinary Incontinence guidelines for women

Stress UI

Stress UI
- First-line treatment for stress or mixed UI should be pelvic floor muscle training (PFMT) lasting at least 3 months.
  - Digitally assess pelvic floor muscle contraction before PFMT.
  - PFMT should consist of at least eight contractions, three times a day.
  - If PFMT is beneficial, continue an exercise programme.
  - During PFMT, do not routinely use:
    - Electrical stimulation; consider it and/or biofeedback in women who cannot actively contract their pelvic floor muscles
    - Biofeedback using perineometry or pelvic floor electromyography.
- Duloxetine:
  - Should not be used as a first-line treatment for stress UI
  - Should not routinely be used as a second-line treatment for stress UI
  - May be offered as an alternative to surgical treatment; counsel women about adverse effects.

Further assessment
- For the few women with pure stress UI multi-channel cystometry is not routinely necessary before primary surgery
- Use multi-channel filling and voiding cystometry before surgery for UI if:
  - There is clinical suspicion of detrusor overactivity, or
  - There has been previous surgery for stress UI or anterior compartment prolapse, or
  - There are symptoms of voiding dysfunction.
- Ambulatory urodynamics or videourodynamics may be considered before surgery for UI in the same circumstances as multi-channel filling and voiding cystometry.

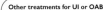

Other treatments for UI or OAB
- Consider desmopressin to reduce troublesome nocturia.
- Consider propiverine to treat frequency of urination in OAB.
- The following are not recommended:
  - Propiverine for the treatment of UI
  - Flavoxate, imipramine and propantheline
  - Systemic hormone-replacement therapy
  - Complementary therapies.

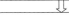

Stress UI
- Discuss the risks and benefits of surgical and non-surgical options. Consider the woman's child-bearing wishes during the discussion
- If conservative treatments have failed, consider:
  - Retropubic mid-urethral tape procedures using a 'bottom-up' approach with macroporous (type 1) polypropylene meshes, open colposuspension or autologous rectus fascial sling
  - synthetic slings using a retropubic 'top-down' or a transobturator foramen approach. Explain the lack of long-term outcome data
  - Intramural bulking agents (glutaraldehyde crosslinked collagen, silicone, carbon-coated zirconium beads, hyaluronic acid/dextran co-polymer). Explain that:
    - Repeat injections may be needed
    - The effect decreases over time
    - The technique is less effective than retropubic suspension or sling.
  - An artificial urinary sphincter if previous surgery has failed.
- The following are not recommended for stress UI:
  - Routine use of laparoscopic colposuspension
  - Synthetic slings using materials other than polypropylene that are not of a macroporous (type 1) construction
  - Anterior colporrhaphy, needle suspensions, paravaginal defect repair and the Marshall-Marchetti-Krantz procedure
  - Autologous fat and polytetrafluoroethylene as intramural bulking agents.

Reproduced with the permission of the Royal College of Obstetricians and Gynaecologists.

6 International Consultation on Incontinence guidelines for women

Initial management of urinary incontinence in women

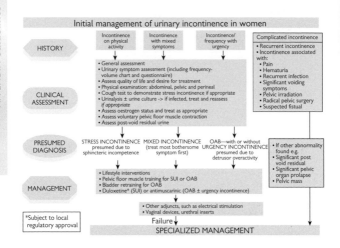

HISTORY

| Incontinence on physical activity | Incontinence with mixed symptoms | Incontinence/frequency with urgency | Complicated incontinence |

Complicated incontinence:
- Recurrent incontinence
- Incontinence associated with:
  - Pain
  - Hematuria
  - Recurrent infection
  - Significant voiding symptoms
  - Pelvic irradiation
  - Radical pelvic surgery
  - Suspected fistual

CLINICAL ASSESSMENT

- General assessment
- Urinary symptom assessment (including frequency-volume chart and questionnaire)
- Assess quality of life and desire for treatment
- Physical examination: abdominal, pelvic and perineal
- Cough test to demonstrate stress incontinence if appropriate
- Urinalysis ± urine culture -> if infected, treat and reassess *if appropriate*
- Assess oestrogen status and treat as appropriate
- Assess voluntary pelvic floor muscle contraction
- Assess post-void residual urine

PRESUMED DIAGNOSIS

STRESS INCONTINENCE presumed due to sphincteric incompetence / MIXED INCONTINENCE (treat most bothersome symptom first) / OAB—with or without URGENCY INCONTINENCE presumed due to detrusor overactivity

- If other abnormality found e.g.
  - Significant post void residual
  - Significant pelvic organ prolapse
  - Pelvic mass

MANAGEMENT

- Lifestyle interventions
- Pelvic floor muscle training for SUI or OAB
- Bladder retraining for OAB
- Duloxetine* (SUI) or antimuscarinic (OAB ± urgency incontinence)

- Other adjuncts, such as electrical stimulation
- Vaginal devices, urethral inserts

Failure ↓

SPECIALIZED MANAGEMENT

*Subject to local regulatory approval

Specialized management of urinary incontinence in women

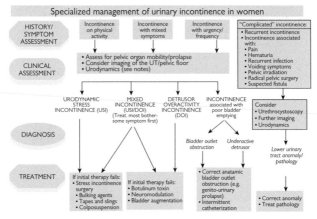

HISTORY/ SYMPTOM ASSESSMENT

| Incontinence on physical activity | Incontinence with mixed symptoms | Incontinence with urgency/frequency | "Complicated" incontinence |

"Complicated" incontinence:
- Recurrent incontinence
- Incontinence associated with:
  - Pain
  - Hematuria
  - Recurrent infection
  - Voiding symptoms
  - Pelvic irradiation
  - Radical pelvic surgery
  - Suspected fistula

CLINICAL ASSESSMENT

- Assess for pelvic organ mobility/prolapse
- Consider imaging of the UT/pelvic floor
- Urodynamics (see notes)

DIAGNOSIS

URODYNAMIC STRESS INCONTINENCE (USI) / MIXED INCONTINENCE (USI/DOI) (Treat. most bothersome symptom first) / DETRUSOR OVERACTIVITY INCONTINENCE (DOI) / INCONTINENCE associated with poor bladder emptying

Bladder outlet obstruction / *Underactive detrusor*

Consider
- Urethrocystoscopy
- Further imaging
- Urodynamics

Lower urinary tract anomaly/ pathology

TREATMENT

If initial therapy fails:
- Stress incontinence surgery
  - Bulking agents
  - Tapes and slings
  - Colposuspension

If initial therapy fails:
- Botulinum toxin
- Neuromodulation
- Bladder augmentation

- Correct anatomic bladder outlet obstruction (e.g. genito-urinary prolapse)
- Intermittent catheterization

- Correct anomaly
- Treat pathology

7 International Consultation on Incontinence guidelines for neurogenic urinary incontinence

Initial management of neurogenic urinary incontinence

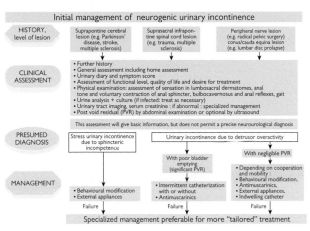

Specialized management of neurogenic urinary incontinence

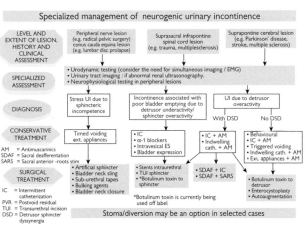

8 International Consultation on Incontinence guidelines for elderly persons

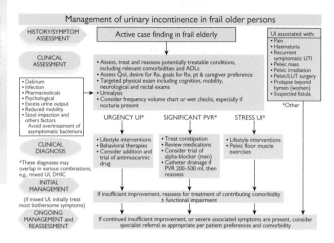

Management of urinary incontinence in frail older persons

Key references

Abrams P, Andersson KE, Birder L, Brubaker L, Cardozo L, Chapple C, et al. (2010). Fourth International Consultation on Incontinence Recommendations of the International Scientific Committee: Evaluation and treatment of urinary incontinence, pelvic organ prolapse, and fecal incontinence. *Neurourol Urodyn*, **29**, 213–40.

Abrams A, Chapple C, Khoury S, Roehrborn C, de la Rosette J (2009). Evaluation and treatment of lower urinary tract symptoms in older men. *J Urol*, **181**, 1779–87.

NICE CG40 (2006). Urinary incontinence: the management of urinary incontinence in women. Available at: http://guidance.nice.org.uk/CG40.

NICE CG97 (2010). The management of lower urinary tract symptoms in men. Available at: http://guidance.nice.org.uk/CG97.